UNASSISTED CHILDBIRTH

UNASSISTED CHILDBIRTH

LAURA KAPLAN SHANLEY

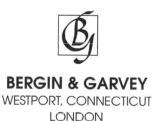

BERGIN & GARVEY
WESTPORT, CONNECTICUT
LONDON

Library of Congress Cataloging-in-Publication Data

Shanley, Laura Kaplan.
    Unassisted childbirth / Laura Kaplan Shanley.
       p.   cm.
    Includes bibliographical references and index.
    ISBN 0–89789–370–0 (alk. paper).—ISBN 0–89789–377–8 (pbk.:
    alk. paper)
    1. Natural childbirth.   I. Title.
    RG661.S48   1994
    618.4'5—dc20   93–5268

British Library Cataloguing in Publication Data is available.

Library of Congress Catalog Card Number: 93–5268
ISBN: 0–89789–370–0
     0–89789–377–8 (pbk.)

First published in 1994

Bergin & Garvey, 88 Post Road West, Westport, CT 06881
An imprint of Greenwood Publishing Group, Inc.

Printed in the United States of America

The paper used in this book complies with the
Permanent Paper Standard issued by the National
Information Standards Organization (Z39.48–1984).

10 9 8 7 6 5 4 3 2 1

Copyright Acknowledgments

Grateful acknowledgment is made to:

Lila Carter, for permission to quote from *Come Gently, Sweet Lucina* (1957) by Patricia Cloyd Carter.

Kathy Lanzalotta and Stephen Lanzalotta, for permission to quote from the newsletter *Two Attune*.

Marilyn Moran, for permission to quote from the newsletter *The New Nativity*, and from her books *Birth and the Dialogue of Love* (1981) and *Happy Birth Days* (1986).

Acknowledgments

This book was actually conceived in 1976 when my soon-to-be husband, David, presented me with a copy of Grantly Dick-Read's *Childbirth without Fear* (1959). A seed was planted the moment I began turning the pages. A new bud emerged with each child to whom I gave birth. And at last, it blossomed into this book.

Aside from my immediate family, I have never come face to face with most of the people who were instrumental in its creation. Many of them I know only by their written words: Jane Roberts, Gerald Heard, and Pat Carter, to name a few. Others I know through numerous letters and phone calls: Marilyn Moran, Kathy Lanzalotta, Rob Butts, and Lynn Flint.

Perhaps my greatest contributors, however, were those who lived with me on a day-to-day basis: my family. John kept me thinking, Willie kept me laughing, Joy kept me company, Michelle kept me dreaming, and David kept me believing. My heartfelt thanks also go out to my parents Herb and Bea Kaplan, my mothers-in-law Elva Shanley and Jeri Fitzgerald, and my sisters Susan Jacobs and Janet Kaplan. My only hope is that in this book I may give back to them, in some way, what they have so generously given to me.

Miracles are nature unimpeded.
—Jane Roberts

Contents

Preface

Someday women will not give birth in hospitals, because they will realize that childbirth is not a disease. They will not pay physicians thousands of dollars to probe them and cut them and tell them what to do. They will not submit themselves to enemas, IVs, fetal monitors, vaginal examinations, or Cesarean sections. Nor will they take the hospitals into their homes, bringing there the well-meaning substitute doctors—the midwives—with their sterilized instruments, rubber gloves, and breathing techniques. For, none of this will be necessary.

Instead, like their animal sisters, women will someday deliver their own babies peacefully and painlessly at home. Women will understand that birth is only dangerous and painful for those who believe it is.

Someday, both women and men will understand that childbirth (and every other event in their lives) is the result of their individual beliefs. They will no longer listen to the voices of officialdom telling them that their lives are beyond their self-conscious control. They will listen instead to the inner authority saying, *"Your life is your own creation. Believe in yourself and you have nothing to fear."*

My goal in writing this book is to help make that someday today.

Introduction

Why should we be content with merely painless childbirth as our norm? Obviously it is our duty to aim at nothing less than perfection, and since we cannot conceive of the perfection of a vitally bodily function so closely related to consciousness as childbirth, unless it is pleasurable, we have no alternative but to set up pleasurable childbirth as the norm, the standard to which we should aspire for all healthy, well-conditioned women.

—Anthony M. Ludivici,
The Truth about Childbirth

In 1976, my husband David and I became aware of the concept that we create our own reality according to our desires, beliefs, and intentions. Undesirable events are neither punishments handed out by an angry God, nor chance happenings that originate from without the self for no apparent reason. They are instead the result of an untrained mind that has not yet become aware of its own abilities.

The following year, after working with our beliefs and success-fully applying this concept to various aspects of our lives, we decided to have a baby. Why, we reasoned, if we are the creators of our lives, should we create anything less than a safe, painless, emotionally and physically fulfilling birth. Furthermore, if birth could actually be this way, why not deliver the baby ourselves?

In August 1978, David delivered (or, more appropriately, "caught") our son John, after a short, easy labor. In 1980, 1982, and 1987, I delivered Willie, Joy, and Michelle respectively, by myself.

Since that time, I've read numerous books and articles about both home and hospital birth. I've realized that much of what we did intuitively is actually recommended by some of the more freethinking childbirth "professionals." I differ from them, however, in that I see no need for their involvement. Medical intervention is based on the belief that childbirth is inherently dangerous. When we choose to believe otherwise, any sort of intervention or assistance becomes unnecessary.

In the course of my studies, I also discovered that, contrary to popular thought, the recent "advances" in medical technology have actually led to an increase in the number of obstetrical problems, rather than a decrease. In countries where women are allowed, or rather allow themselves, to give birth more naturally and with fewer interventions, the outcome for both mothers and babies is remarkably good.

Most women in this culture have been led to believe they are incapable of delivering their own babies. Even most feminists, who look back in horror to the days when women were told they must rely on others (generally men) for their emotional and financial support, still do not hesitate in labor to turn themselves over to a person of "authority." The notion that women are self-reliant, independent, competent human beings has not, at this point in time, been fully applied to the act of giving birth. Childbirth—an event that should ideally reinforce a woman's sense of power and autonomy—has now become a painful, dangerous ordeal that often ends up reinforcing the belief she is indeed a helpless, dependent child herself.

Many women simply do not want to deliver their own babies. They enjoy the presence of others in all aspects of their lives. My intention is not to dissuade them. I thoroughly support women in whatever way they choose to give birth. If a woman decides to share her birth with others, however, it should be because she chooses to—not because she feels she has to, out of fear of pain and problems.

Therefore, I present unassisted childbirth not as a way childbirth *should* be done, but rather as a way it *can* be done. Giving birth without medical assistance was a life-changing, thoroughly fulfilling experience for me, and I feel compelled to share my story with others who may have found the technocratic model of birth less than satisfying. (*Webster's* defines technocracy as "management of society by technical experts.")

We create our own reality. When the world understands this concept fully, then war, sickness, poverty, and unhappiness will no longer be a part of our experience. The world, however, is made up of individuals. It is up to each one of us to cast off our doubts and fears and begin to believe in our own abilities. What better place to start than with the birth of a baby?

UNASSISTED CHILDBIRTH

Chapter One

We've Come a Long Way—Or Have We?

The more civilized the people, the more the pain of labor appears to become intensified.

—Grantly Dick-Read, M.D.
Childbirth without Fear

I remember listening, as a child, to my mother talk about her experiences in labor. She smiled as she told me of the shaving of the pubic hair, the enema, the "slight" pain of the contractions, the epidural, and the episiotomy. But I could feel the fear in her voice. Labor had not been easy for her; and whatever had been good about it could be attributed, in her mind, to modern medicine.

"Can you believe," she said to me once, "that, up until a hundred years ago, women had to go through labor without any sort of medication?"

"What did they do?" I asked, horrified.

"They suffered," she replied.

I don't recall hearing anything pleasant about childbirth from anyone else either. I did hear several horror stories, however, from "friends" and relatives. "I spent my entire pregnancy leaning over a toilet. Then to top it all off, I was in labor for four days," said one. "It was the worst experience I've ever had. I screamed at my husband that he was never going to touch me again!" said another.

Somehow the women had managed to survive, as most women have throughout the centuries. It was just part of the curse of being a woman—moodiness, menstrual cramps, labor pains, and the hot flashes of menopause. No one questioned it, or so I thought. That was just the way things were.

When I was about eight or nine years old, I remember watching a movie on television that left in my mind a lasting impression concerning the trials of pregnancy. In the movie, a woman suddenly fainted in the midst of doing her housework. After an examination by the kindly old family doctor, she was informed that she was with child. Pulling her husband aside, the doctor whispered, "Better have the little lady take it easy now that she's in a delicate condition" (or words to that effect).

"So that's what happens when you're pregnant," I thought. *"You become weak and you faint. You throw up for a few months and then go through hours or maybe days of excruciating pain—and for what? Some dumb kid! No thanks."* I don't remember even considering motherhood. The episiotomy alone gave me nightmares. It didn't occur to me at the time that perhaps those attitudes toward childbirth, and womanhood in general, had something to do with the outcome of women's labors.

Not much has changed in the past thirty years as far as the "official" version of childbirth goes. Movies and television—our most influential media—continue to do their part to perpetuate the beliefs that pregnancy is a disease characterized by vomiting, backaches, strange cravings, and swollen ankles, and that childbirth is a painful, dangerous ordeal requiring the direction and assistance of a skilled professional.

In the 1970s, an episode of the popular TV series *M*A*S*H* showed a Korean woman crying and screaming while giving birth to twins. Luckily she was in the good hands of Hawkeye Pierce who, in the tradition of the old Wild West doctors, shoved a piece of gauze into her mouth for her to bite on.

In the 1989 hit movie *Look Who's Talking*, Kirstie Alley's character also screamed her way through labor. It was all very "funny," of course, but everyone was relieved when the doctor finally shot her up with a big dose of Demerol.

In the sequel, *Look Who's Talking Too*, the doctor "determined" that baby #2 was in "distress," so he ordered that a Cesarean be done. Immediately following the birth, the baby was taken away from the mother and placed in an isolette for "observation." At that point, Roseanne Arnold as the voice of the baby said, "First a bad birth; now this. Life sucks!" Unfortunately, that part of the movie was accurate. A traumatic birth leaves a lasting impression on an infant's mind, setting the tone for future experiences.

In 1992, TV's Murphy Brown gave birth in one of the most watched episodes of any TV series ever. Of course, she too screamed in pain with every contraction. Unlike Kirstie Alley's character, however, she did not receive medication but endured the pain as any good martyr would. Dan Quayle need not worry. Whatever single women the story line may have inspired to have babies out of wedlock must surely have changed their minds after listening to Murphy's blood-curdling screams.

These are the images of childbirth that surround us in this country today. We are told we may choose between drugging ourselves and our unborn children, submitting to surgery in the form of a C-section, and panting and pushing our way through endless hours of painful contractions in what some people call "natural childbirth."

I contend that panting, pushing, and pain are not natural at all. There is another way of giving birth. One has only to observe the average house cat in labor to see true natural childbirth in action. She has no manuals to read or "experts" to tell her what to do. She is not shaved or given enemas and episiotomies, and yet she gives birth gracefully and easily.

According to Purina's *Handbook of Cat Care* (1981), it is precisely this lack of intervention that allows the cat to give birth as easily as she does. The book advises the cat owner to pet the cat

> reassuringly and leave her on her own. She may stay in the box; on the other hand, don't be surprised if she doesn't. The best thing to do at this point is to do nothing. Keep quiet and do not attempt to help her—it's her problem. Mother nature usually takes over at this point and it is amazing to see how she goes about doing what comes naturally. (Purina 1981:58)

Desmond Morris, author of *Cat Watching*, states, "Most female cats are amazingly good midwives and need no help from their human owners" (1986:89). Anthony M. Ludivici reports in *The Truth about Childbirth* (1938) that his cat not only gave birth easily; she actually purred while doing it.

Not only cats, however, give birth easily. Obstetrician and child-birth educator Robert Bradley writes in *Husband-coached Childbirth* about growing up on a farm and witnessing numerous farm animal births: "The birth processes I witnessed in these many creatures were attended with no objective evidence of pain or suffering. The opposite was true. The animal mother's eyes were radiant with joy and happiness" (1965:8).

The same scenario also occurs in undomesticated animals. In an article in *Scientific American*, Dr. William F. Windle wrote about rhesus monkeys giving birth:

> Most monkey births occur at night, as is the case with human beings. Labor is short: an hour or less. The female squats and drops the infant on the ground. During the delivery most of the blood in the placenta passes to the infant and, as the uterus continues to contract after birth, the placenta is ex-pelled. (Windle 1969:77)

Many people have heard stories about women in less techno-logically developed cultures giving birth quickly and easily as well. A friend of mine who was actually in Korea in the 1960s said he saw a pregnant Korean woman working in the rice fields one day. She walked over to the edge of the field, squatted down, caught her baby, strapped it to her back and was back picking rice minutes later. (All, mind you, without the help of Alan Alda!) Several people watched the birth from a distance, but no one helped or interfered in any way. She did it quietly, by herself.

Midwife Penny Armstrong writes about birth in an Amish community in her book *A Wise Birth*:

> I was struck by the casual, comfortable movements of the women laboring in their kitchen and giving birth among the quilts. Having based much of my assessment of myself as a practitioner on my ability to respond swiftly and accurately

to emergency situations, I was undone by the infrequency of the need for me to display my masterly strokes. Birth appeared to be another animal out in the country. Labors were shorter than I was accustomed to. Pain appeared to be less severe. Cuts and tears fewer. Hemorrhage controllable. Babies did not need my suctioning devices or my tubes pressed down their throats; they gurgled when they were born and began to breathe. Their mothers took them to their breasts and nursed without much complication. If problems did arise anytime during a birth, most of them appeared to resolve themselves in short order. I had an eerie sense of unreality. The births had not only power, but grace and simplicity. (Armstrong and Feldman 1990:34)

People who have observed births in tribal cultures also describe it as being similar to animal births. In *The Paleolithic Prescription*, S. Boyd Eaton writes about a typical birth in a !Kung San village in Africa's Kalahari Desert:

A woman feels the initial stages of labor and makes no comment, leaves the village quietly when birth seems imminent—taking along, if necessary, a young child—walks a few hundred yards, finds an area in the shade, clears it, arranges a soft bed of leaves, and gives birth, while squatting or lying on her side—on her own. Unusual even for other hunters and gatherers, solo birth for !Kung San women is nevertheless an ideal: 35% of women attain it by their third birth and the majority do on subsequent births. Showing no fear and not screaming out, they believe enhances the ease and safety of delivery. (Eaton, Shostak, and Konner 1988:240)

Judith Goldsmith relays similar stories of birth in *Childbirth Wisdom from the World's Oldest Societies* (1990). Goldsmith compiled the accounts of scientists, anthropologists, and historians who had observed tribal births over the past four hundred years. She makes many references to the fact that tribal women often delivered their own babies.

There were numerous societies where women gave birth with no assistance at all. Among the Chukchee of Siberia, for example, where babies were born with little trouble, the birthing woman attended completely to her own needs and those of her newborn infant. She cut the umbilical cord and disposed of the placenta herself. During the birth, the only other person present was an older woman, who aided the mother in the case of absolute necessity. . . . The Fulani woman of Africa also birthed without expecting any assistance, catching the infant as it was born in her own hands. (Goldsmith 1990:23–24)

In 1791 a traveler among the Guinea women of South America noted that, if an Indian woman went into labor while on "the march," she simply stepped aside, caught the baby, and ran in haste after the others. In West Africa around 1800 a doctor observed that a delivery was often conducted without a single attendant or without its being known to anyone.

An English settler observed a New Zealand woman working in the fields in 1869. The woman walked a short distance alone, gave birth to her child, and returned to work two hours later. Two hundred years ago, if a North American native woman went into labor while traveling by canoe, she would ask to be put ashore, go into the woods alone, return shortly with her baby, and resume paddling. Among the Maria Gonds of India, Goldsmith writes, there are no midwives. "It is assumed that the mother will do everything for herself" (Goldsmith 1990:24).

One of Goldsmith's more interesting stories concerning tribal birth comes from Livingston Jones who observed the Tlinget women of Alaska. Most Tlinget women, he writes, suffer very little if any during birth. Some of them actually give birth while sleeping. (Ludivici writes there are numerous recorded instances of women going into labor while asleep and waking to find they have given birth.) Another Tlinget observer noted that the women give birth painlessly and quickly and return to their work within half an hour.

Goldsmith states that, although infant mortality rates may have been high in some of the tribal cultures she studied, the deaths generally occurred within the first year of life, primarily due to malnutrition. The births themselves were seldom fatal to either mother or child. A visitor to North America in 1641 wrote that the natives were rarely sick in childbirth, nor did any of them die either during or after the birth. Another observer noted in 1884 that accidents in childbirth rarely occurred. A physician who spent eight years living with the Canadian Indians reported he knew of no deaths from childbirth. People who observed tribal births in Fiji, Uganda, and Argentina also claimed that death during childbirth was rare.

Complications normally associated with pregnancy and child-birth are usually quite uncommon in tribal societies. A man who observed the Arikara of North Dakota during the 1930s noted there was no tubal or abdominal pregnancy, no placenta previa (a situation where the placenta separates prematurely and blocks the entrance to the birth canal), no eclampsia (convulsions), and no premature birth (except in the case of an accident). Phlebitis (inflammation of a vein) only occurred after tribal women became exposed to more "progressive" cultures.

In *Spiritual Midwifery* (1978), Ina May Gaskin writes that vomiting during pregnancy—a common occurrence in our society—is rare among the native people of the world.

Although it is not without its problems, overall pregnancy and birth both in animals and in tribal cultures appears to be much easier and less painful than it is in modern, technologically developed societies. What, we must ask ourselves, can account for the differences?

From a physical standpoint, animals and tribal women are generally in much better shape than most Western women are. They continue to be active right up until they give birth. Exercise alone, however, cannot account for the dramatic discrepancies. If this were true, American female athletes would give birth quickly and easily; and studies show this is not the case.

Physiologically, there is no difference between a tribal woman and a Western woman, and little difference between humans and other mammals. Therefore, if we are to understand the vast differences in births, we must examine the method in which the deliveries occur and the psychological differences between animals, tribal women, and modern Western women.

Psychological historian Gerald Heard writes about the evolution of self-consciousness in his book *The Five Ages of Man* (1963). Since the completion of our physical evolution, Heard says, we have been evolving psychologically. Contrary to what many "scientists" believe, there is a design and purpose to this evolution. The purpose is to create a self-conscious reasoning human being who can understand both herself and her nonphysical source. By nonphysical source, he's not referring to some nebulous God in the sky, but rather to a highly evolved, multidimensional, loving, and creative consciousness that is behind and within all life.

In order to develop a self-conscious personality, we have temporarily had to "forget" our spiritual origins and focus exclusively on what has come to be called the "ego." We are much more than simply our egos, however. We are multidimensional beings—little gods, in a sense—endowed with all of the characteristics of our Creator. Heard claims that our ego is now sufficiently developed that we may once again become aware of our inner selves.

In becoming self-conscious, Heard writes, we have developed unnatural beliefs in fear, shame, and guilt. These beliefs manifest themselves in a multitude of physical and psychological problems. The fear, he says, stems from our ignorance of ourselves and our world. The shame and guilt stem from our belief that we have somehow "sinned" by "eating from the tree of knowledge," that is, becoming self-conscious. In a way, we believe we are not quite as acceptable as the animals who have remained in their pre-self-conscious state. It is true that animals are more in tune with the universe. They lack, however, the ability to comprehend themselves fully, and so are limited in their experiences.

As human beings, we can have the best of both worlds. We can retain our self-conscious personalities while at the same time becoming aware of our inner selves. To do this we must first rid ourselves of the unnatural emotions of fear, shame, and guilt, for they are like clouds preventing us from seeing who we are and what we're capable of doing. This can be accomplished through love, forgiveness, and understanding.

True religion was designed to eliminate these undesirable emotions and reunite the separated self-conscious ego with its inner self. Most organized religions today fail to do either one. They not only perpetuate beliefs in fear, shame, and guilt, rather than alleviate them; they also encourage dependence on external authority rather than internal authority.

Individuals themselves have little knowledge of this process. Therefore, the majority of people in intellectually developed societies are both psychologically and physically unhealthy. Because they are unaware of the existence of the inner self, they are unable to utilize the constant help and guidance that is available to them. Animals, on the other hand, have little sense of themselves as individuals, but they intuitively avail themselves of this guidance.

The tribal woman, in a sense, has a consciousness that lies between that of the animal and that of the modern Western woman. Her births are successful for several reasons. She has not yet developed beliefs in fear, shame, and guilt, and therefore is free from their devastating consequences. In addition to this, like the cat in the closet, she is generally left alone. This privacy not only allows her body to perform its task easily because it is unhampered by outside intervention, it also allows her psychologically to reconnect with her inner self. The inner self speaks to her—just as it does to the Western woman—through her dreams, impulses, and intuition. The difference is, she listens.

The Western woman, for the most part, does not believe this inner self exists. Even if it does, she has little faith in its ability to help her in childbirth. Therefore she turns herself over to the medical profession, and that is where the problems begin.

> Culture has been doing its best to destroy the safety and beauty of normal childbirth for many generations. It has tried hard to demonstrate the wonders of science upon the greatest miracle of nature. It has failed to understand the simplicity of truth and unhesitatingly introduced the complexity of falsehood. (Dick-Read 1959:284)

Chapter Two

The Dangers of Medical Intervention

obstetrician: n., from obstare—to stand in the way
—*Webster's New Collegiate Dictionary*

More and more, research confirms the fact that intervening in the act of childbirth causes serious problems for both the mother and the baby. Not only does the presence of numerous doctors, nurses, and hospital equipment make it difficult for the woman to relax and slip into the type of consciousness necessary for a baby to be born easily; the actual physical intervention of the doctor generally makes it virtually impossible.

Often a woman will say, "Thank God I was in the hospital when I gave birth. There were complications, but the doctor saved my baby's life." What she may not understand is that the interference by the doctor and the nursing staff, from the moment she entered the hospital, may have actually caused the "complications" in the first place.

Still, safety is the primary reason most women give for turning themselves over to physicians when they're in labor. Images of women bleeding to death or coming down with strange diseases still flash through the minds of many women.

In reality, women rarely bled to death or came down with diseases until *after* they began submitting themselves to outside intervention. Hemorrhaging after giving birth, Judith Goldsmith writes in *Childbirth Wisdom* (1990), was quite uncommon until midwives in prehospital Europe began tugging on umbilical cords in an attempt to remove a placenta that had not yet been expelled.

The situation only worsened when women began delivering in hospitals. Howard W. Haggard, M.D., writes in *Devils, Drugs, and Doctors* (1929) that laboring women were often placed in the same hospital bed with individuals infected with malaria, typhoid, diphtheria, syphilis, and a myriad of other diseases. Generally, he claims, corpses would lie in the bed for at least twenty-four hours before being removed.

Childbed fever, which killed thousands of women in hospital wards, was found to have been caused by the doctors themselves. Suzanne Arms writes in *Immaculate Deception*,

> "Physicians" of all kinds—students, barbers, butchers, and (in some areas) shepherds and hog gelders—worked on women in labor as part of their medical training. Often they would arrive with their hands still bloody from dissecting cadavers of diseased patients, and would then insert their hands far up into the birth canals of laboring women, infecting one and all with the germs that remained on their unwashed skin. So the "doctor" himself, sporting a bloodied apron as a badge of his "profession," became the carrier of the very disease he was supposed to cure, and childbed fever became the scourge of Europe for more than two centuries. If the woman had anything left of the matter-of-fact sensibilities in birth of her primitive ancestor, she was now consumed with abject terror. (Arms 1975:17–18)

In the 1800s, writes Jessica Mitford in *The American Way of Birth* (1992), thousands of women used to suffer from a disease known as "vesicovaginal fistulae," tears in the walls between the vagina and the bladder that occurred during childbirth. Often it was found to have been the result of a badly botched forceps delivery. Women afflicted with the disease not only became lifelong invalids, but were social outcasts as well. The tears caused uncontrollable leakage of the bladder, and the smell was said to be intolerable.

Today we have more sophisticated means of intervention. What follows is a brief explanation of some of the routine procedures carried out in most hospitals.

INDUCTION

Approximately 20 percent of hospital births are a result of induction. A woman is usually induced when she does not go into labor within two weeks of her estimated due date. Studies show, however, that about 50 percent of women who were assumed to have gone beyond their due date had actually not done so. In fact, Carl Jones writes in *Mind over Labor* (1987) that the estimated due date is accurate only 5 percent of the time.

Many women who have been induced claim that, according to the date of their last period, they knew they were not overdue. The opinions of pregnant women, however, are generally not considered to be as scientific or accurate as a sonogram (ultrasound), which supposedly shows how far along a woman is in her pregnancy.

Most physicians rely heavily on ultrasound tests when determining a woman's due date, even though—according to an article in the *Rocky Mountain News* (Denver, Colo. December 1, 1992)—more than a third of the facilities that perform the tests do not meet the guidelines established by many medical groups. "Currently there is no established accreditation program for facilities providing these exams. Our study shows a significant number may be substandard in quality," said Michael Clair of Fox Chase Cancer Center and Jeanes Hospital in Philadelphia.

Consequently, many women are induced or C-sectioned only to give birth to a premature baby. In *Confessions of a Medical Heretic*, Robert S. Mendelsohn, M.D., writes, "A labor induced by the doctor can end up a Cesarean delivery because a baby that's not ready to be born will naturally show more distress on fetal monitors, distress at being summoned prematurely" (1979:54).

Pitocin, the drug used to induce labor, makes the contractions quite painful, so anesthesia is often given to reduce the pain. Anesthesia tends to slow the course of labor, so more Pitocin must then be given.

According to childbirth educator Sheila Kitzinger, babies who are born after a drug-induced labor are three times more likely to have trouble breathing at birth. This, Kitzinger writes, may be totally unnecessary. In *Birth at Home* (1979), she cites one study in which it was discovered that an electronic breast pump used for fifteen minutes on each breast could actually induce labor in 71 percent of women. In another study, it was found that nipple stimulation could induce labor in approximately forty-five minutes, as compared with ninety minutes for Pitocin. This is because oxytocin—the hormone that stimulates uterine contractions—is naturally produced by the body when the nipples are stimulated. Pitocin is artificial oxytocin.

> They induced me and one minute later the baby's heart rate dropped and never (again) reached its normal rate of 145. The doctor had lied—the pitocin had drastically affected my baby's heart rate. I should have removed the IV right then but I still believed that the doctors wouldn't do anything dangerous. (*Two Attune* 1992, #8:4)

> It should be emphasized that in all cases of induced labor— and this is true with other interferences as well—it is not the mother, nor the doctor, but *the baby* whose delicate system must correct the effects of such interference as soon as extrauterine life begins. Since many of the infant's vital organs are only beginning to function at the time of birth . . . such artificial effects as change in acid balance, respiratory sluggishness, or disalignment of parietal bones [all of what can occur when labor is artificially induced], are extraordinary burdens to place on such a physiologically innocent beginner of independent life. (Arms 1975:58)

INSISTENCE ON THE SUPINE POSITION DURING LABOR AND DELIVERY

Most women in this country are told that the safest place to labor and deliver is in bed. Research shows that often the opposite is true. Katherine Camacho Carr, a certified nurse midwife, conducted a cross-cultural study of birthing positions in 1980. She concluded that lying on the back and lying in the Lamaze position (on the back in a propped position) are the worst possible positions for the laboring woman. In fact, they may actually prolong labor.

Writing in *Family Practice News*, Dr. Roberto Caldeyro-Barcia, past president of the International Federation of Obstetricians and Gynecologists, agrees: "Except for being hanged by the feet, the supine position is the worst conceivable position for labor and delivery" (1975:11). Not only is the mother unable to utilize the natural gravitational force; the lower aorta is compressed, resulting in reduced blood circulation in the mother and reduced blood supply to the baby.

The bed itself may not always be conducive to a quick and easy labor. Simply getting up and walking around has been found to stimulate contractions more effectively than Pitocin. Sheila Kitzinger cites one study in which it was found that women who were allowed to walk around while in labor had shorter labors, less need for pain-relieving drugs, and more regular heartbeats of their babies than women who were forced to stay in bed. Perhaps it would do physicians well to read Purina's *Handbook of Cat Care*, which states, "Let her walk around [while in labor] and do not insist that she stay in her box" (1981:58).

Studies have shown that, when women are free to choose their position for labor and delivery, they rarely choose to lie down. Physician Michel Odent reported that of the one thousand deliveries occurring one year in his hospital in Pithiviers, France, only *two* of the women chose to give birth lying down (Balaskas 1992). No other culture in the world (aside from those who have been recently influenced by Western beliefs) delivers in the supine position.

It's funny—it seems so normal to lie down in labor—just to be in the hospital seems to mean "to lie down." But as soon as I did, I felt that I had lost something. I felt defeated. And it seems to me now that my lying down tacitly permitted the Demerol, or maybe entailed it. And the Demerol entailed the pitocin, and the pitocin entailed the Cesarean. It was as if, in laying down my body as I was told to, I also laid down my autonomy and my right to self-direction. (David-Floyd 1992:87)

I was told if I did get out of bed I'd somehow compromise the
delivery. The baby's head would fall on the cord or something. I
just felt so much alone and hopeless. It was out of control. . . . I
thought, "This is not what I wanted it to be like." (Abbott 1992b)

Allowing gravity to help descent of the baby's head by keeping
out of bed and moving around can almost always avoid prolapse
of the umbilical cord. (Kitzinger 1979:39)[emphasis added]

THE IV

IVs are inserted into the arms of approximately 80 percent of all
laboring women after they are admitted to the hospital. Doctors in
this country believe a woman should fast during labor just in case
she must undergo surgery. Hydrating fluids may therefore be
given intravenously to sustain a woman undergoing a long labor.
IVs are also used to give anesthesia, analgesia, Pitocin, and fluids
for emergency surgical intervention.

There is no research to show there is any benefit to placing an
IV in a woman's arm before there is an actual emergency. Some
women develop infections at the site of the IV. There is also a chance
that too much fluid can enter the woman's body tissues, which may
result in electrolyte imbalance, cardiac arrhythmia, and pulmonary
edema (fluid in the lungs).

Depriving a woman of nourishment during labor can be dangerous in and of itself. Research has shown that lack of food may
slow down the progression of labor as well as result in there being
less oxygen going to the unborn baby.

As Robbie Davis-Floyd—author of *Birth as an American Rite of
Passage* (1992)—states, placing an IV in a woman's arm is above all a
symbolic gesture designed to reinforce the concept that women are
totally dependent on physicians, machines, and institutions for the
successful outcome of their labors. The intravenous tubes are a symbolic umbilical cord; and the woman, a helpless dependent infant.

SHAVING OF THE PUBIC AREA

More than half of the American women giving birth in hospitals
are routinely shaved—supposedly to reduce the risk of infection.

Research has shown that women who have been shaved actually have a greater rate of infection than those who have not, in part because nurses have been known occasionally to cut a woman while shaving her.

Psychotherapist Gayle Peterson believes that shaving of the pubic hair, as well as draping, enemas, and routine episiotomies, are unrecognized attempts to hide the fact that birth is sexual. Not only are they unnecessary; they make a woman feel demeaned. Author Pat Carter agrees. In *Come Gently, Sweet Lucina* she writes,

> [Pubic hair] is our badge of maturity. A woman feels naked and babyfied without it, and this is one time that she should feel quite grown up and confident. . . . It was the symbol of growing up, and though we may think we have lost its meaning with the passing years, we haven't really. . . . [Shaving a woman in labor] is an unnatural act. It is an affront to the body that causes rebellion no matter what conscious submission there is. (Carter 1957:260–262)

ENEMAS

Once again, more than half of all women are given enemas in labor. There is no evidence to prove there is any medical benefit to receiving one. Doctors usually claim they shorten labor and reduce the chances of neonatal infection due to feces contamination. However, in a study done in 1981 involving 274 birthing women randomly assigned to enema and no-enema groups, there was no difference in rates of infection or length of labor. Many women find enemas to be extremely irritating to the rectal tissues. If a woman is relaxed, she will naturally empty her bowels.

> The enema was the single most painful part of Johnathan's birth. (Davis-Floyd 1992:85)

> I still do not believe that either forceps or anesthesia would have been necessary, or my son lamed, had I been spared the enema and other silly "prepping.". . . I had no pain intense enough to call true suffering until the attendants had their way with my body. (Carter 1957:263)

AMNIOTOMY

An amniotomy is the artificial breaking of the bag of waters by the doctor or nurse. It is done to almost all women in an attempt to induce labor, speed up the contractions, or apply an electrode to a baby's head when using a fetal monitor.

However, the pressure from the amniotic sack helps to dilate the cervix, and some studies show that performing an amniotomy may actually prolong labor. The natural descent of the bag of waters also helps to stretch a woman's perineum slowly. Therefore, prematurely rupturing the bag often leads to the performing of an episiotomy.

The amniotic fluid protects the baby's head. So, rupturing the membranes can cause serious problems for the baby as well. Not only does the baby's head receive the full force of the contractions because there is no cushion there to protect it, but the umbilical cord may be compressed causing the baby to be denied necessary oxygen. Amniotomies have also been shown to increase the rate of infection for the mother, as well as the rate of C-sections.

The doctor insisted that breaking my water would really hurry things along. It really hurt to have it done—it was tough and not ready to be broken. The doctor was rough and impatient—I later learned he wanted to catch a football game. (*Two Attune* 1992, #8:4)

FETAL MONITORS

At most hospitals, more than two-thirds of the women in labor are hooked up to a fetal monitor, supposedly so that the doctor may monitor the unborn baby's heart rate. If it is an internal monitor, the baby's scalp is actually pierced with a small screw. The use of a monitor makes it almost impossible for a woman to get up and walk around or take a bath or a shower, all of which are helpful in labor.

Studies have shown that the use of fetal monitors has increased the rate of C-sections. At the first sign of fetal distress (according to the monitor), a doctor may simply order a C-section be done. Edward H. Hon, researcher, professor, and inventor of the electronic fetal monitor said at the "Crisis in Obstetrics—Management of Labor" conference,

Most women in labor are much better off at home than in the hospital with the EFM. Most obstetricians don't understand the monitor. They're dropping the knife with each drop in the fetal heart rate. The C-section is considered as a rescue mission of the baby by the white knight, but actually you've assaulted the mother. (Young and Shearer 1987)

Often it has been found that it is the machine itself that is causing the distress, which it then picks up. Yvonne Brackbill writes in *Birth Trap: The Legal Low-down on High-tech Obstetrics*, "Many mothers leave the hospital firmly convinced that electronic monitoring saved their babies from otherwise certain death caused by cord prolapse when in fact it was the monitor (and prerequisite amniotomy) that caused the prolapse in the first place" (Brackbill, Rice, and Young 1984:11).

Some women experience pain when the electrode is inserted into their cervix, and many wonder what the baby must be feeling. Occasionally a monitor lead leaves a permanent scar on a baby's head.

DRUGS

In most hospitals 80–95 percent of all women in labor are given either analgesia, anesthesia, or both. Analgesia is given for pain relief; and anesthesia, to block sensation. Their use may result in the following:

- a slowdown of labor, requiring additional drugs to speed things up
- a drop in the mother's blood pressure, with life-threatening consequences for both the mother and the baby
- the elimination of the pleasurable sensations of birth
- unresponsiveness of both the mother and the baby after the birth
- inability of the mother to push the baby out, resulting in a forceps delivery
- head and neck aches for the mother that may last several weeks

- breathing and sucking difficulties for the baby
- dulling of the mind and the body, resulting in the inability of the mother and the baby to bond after birth
- vomiting and inhaling of the fluids, resulting in death for the mother
- impaired muscular, visual, and neural development of the baby
- permanent brain damage and mental retardation of the baby
- infant death

Dr. Doris Haire, D.M.S., past president of the International Childbirth Education Association, believes that a large proportion of brain-injured and learning-disabled children are the result of obstetric drugs administered to women in labor. In *The Cultural Warping of Childbirth* she writes, "Recent research makes it evident that obstetrical medication must play a role in our staggering incidence of neurological impairment" (1972:7).

The American Academy of Pediatrics states that no drug has been found to be safe for the baby in utero. In fact, Helen Wessel writes in *Natural Childbirth and the Christian Family* (1963) that 60 percent of the infant deaths in the United States are attributable to lack of sufficient oxygen during birth, partly because of the improper use of drugs. She also writes that anesthetic deaths are now ranked as one of the leading causes of maternal mortality.

I was talked into a shot that "would take the edge off" the contractions. I received a heavy dose of Demerol that reduced my brave determination to tears and a feeling of doom. My husband watched it all and was helpless. I was made to push when I didn't feel ready. This caused blood vessels to burst all over my face. This was done in the presence of an impatient, angry-looking doctor whom I had dreaded seeing the most out of the three doctors who have a racket going on in our small town. Numerous nurses were passing through. We were then told that Robby's head was too large and that I would have to have a spinal and that he would have to be delivered with forceps. The fact that Robby was crowning and that Roger could see his hair made no difference. It must have been a mad rush to get that shot in before my body could deliver the child. I felt nothing more of my body. I got to hold my child for a full two minutes as I was wheeled to my room, and this was with me on my belly being admonished *not* to raise my head because of the spinal. I'm not sure if I've ever felt worse for I didn't get Robby back until 8 hours later. (*New Nativity* 1977, #44:1)

INSISTENCE ON PUSHING

It is a little known fact that, aside from a slight push or two in the last seconds of labor, pushing is not necessary or even desirable for the laboring woman. The saying, "Don't push the river; it flows by itself," definitely applies to labor.

Nancy Tatje-Broussard writes in her article "Second Stage Labor: You Don't Have to Push," "The birth process need not be a pushing affair. It can be a gentle unfolding in harmony with the natural rhythms of life" (1990:78).

Tatje-Broussard began studying the concept of pushing after an older friend of hers shared her story of a medicated flat-on-your-back birth twenty years earlier. The friend had been given general anesthesia, which had rendered her unconscious through most of her labor; but she woke up in time to see her daughter's head emerging. Quickly she called to the nurses who were playing cards at a nearby table.

Tatje-Broussard wondered, if women were able to give birth easily while unconscious, why must they exert tremendous effort while awake? She found that, up until the 1920s, women were not instructed to push during the second stage of labor. (The second stage is the time between the full dilation of the cervix and the delivery of the baby.) Around the 1920s, doctors "determined" that the second stage was dangerous to the unborn baby. Pushing, they hoped, would get the baby out faster. At one time, mothers were even told to begin pushing at the onset of labor.

By the mid-1950s, many people had begun to realize the importance of relaxation during the first stage of labor. However, the second stage was, and continues to be, associated with great physical effort. Doctors, nurses, midwives, and "birth coaches" often encourage a woman to push even when she has no impulse to do so.

By the 1980s, scientific evidence showed that the second stage of labor is not dangerous for the baby, but actually helps to stimulate her digestive, eliminatory, and respiratory systems. Pushing can, in fact, be dangerous to both the mother and the baby. When a woman is pushing, she is holding her breath. Oxygen is therefore not going to her uterus—which makes contracting more difficult and painful. It is also not going to her baby. This can lead to a drop in the fetal heart rate and possible brain damage.

Susan McKay agrees. In her paper "Humanizing Birth in a Technological Society" she writes, "Urging a woman to push harder and longer may, in fact, make things worse as the baby's head and umbilical cord are compressed through the mother's intensive effort, leading to (heart rate) decelerations and fetal hypoxia (oxygen deprivation)" (quoted in Davis-Floyd 1992:117).

Tearing of the perineum is more common for women who have pushed over a long period of time. And studies show that pushing does not necessarily get a baby out faster anyway.

In her article "Childbirth the Amish Way," midwife and author Ina May Gaskin wrote about a birth she attended in an Amish community.

> Just as soon as there was any sign of pushing the baby was crowning. The only sign of her pushing was a slight catch of her breath. She did not make a sound or grimace. Eighteen other births had obviously taught her how to let her uterus do the work while the rest of her took it as easy as possible. (Gaskin 1987:70)

Jan Fletcher told of her labor experience in a *Mothering* magazine letter titled "No More Professional Pushers."

> My first birthing experience was accompanied by a frantic chorus of "Push! Push! Push!" for at least 30 minutes. Being an inexperienced "birther," I took their exhortations seriously. . . . Five people were yelling at me to push, and in my efforts to appease this throng, I pushed so hard that I broke by tailbone. For my second birthing, I made up my mind that

I wasn't going to push at all. If the baby took a while to come out, so be it. Sure enough, the second birth was also accompanied by a chorus of "Push! Push! Push!"—only this time I ignored it. Breathing quietly, relaxing, and hesitating ever so slightly with each breath was all it took. Jessica came out leaving my tailbone in one piece and thereby sparing me six weeks of postpartum pain. (Fletcher 1988:12)

Giving birth is not unlike having a bowel movement. In a normal bowel movement, one allows the body to do its work. Once the feces has entered the rectum, only a slight push is necessary to excrete it. The concept that labor is "hard work! The hardest work I've ever done in my life" (as said one woman) is simply a fallacy. Pat Carter believes, in fact, that neither the woman nor her uterus need to work hard to produce a baby.

It only takes a little bit of effort from the fundus to send a baby merrily and successfully on its way, provided pain inhibition has not set up opposition to its efforts. Little, if any, more power than the walls of the colon have to exert to perform its function of ejection—actually less power than it takes to sneeze. (Carter 1957:257)

On a more aesthetically pleasing level, giving birth can be compared to painting a picture or having an orgasm. It is more a matter of allowing it to happen, rather than making it happen.

True creativity cannot be forced to conform to society's unnatural time constraints. The insistence on pushing in labor is simply a reflection of our cultural attitude that force and haste are superior to trust and patience.

AUGMENTATION

Augmentation is the administering of drugs in an attempt to speed up labor. When a labor is not progressing quickly enough according to the "Friedman curve," doctors often resort to Pitocin. The Friedman curve is supposedly based on the average number of hours that most women labor. Even Dr. Emmanuel E. Friedman himself, however, does not believe his findings are absolute.

"There is no magic number of hours," he says, "beyond which labor should not continue. . . . [The curve] is being abused more than it is being used appropriately" (Young and Shearer 1987). (He deems intervening with a Cesarean for prolonged labor "unthinkable.")

Pitocin, as with any drug, has negative side effects. Besides making the contractions more painful, it has been found to increase the rate of jaundice in newborns as well as cause fetal distress, mental retardation, placental separation, and rupturing of the uterus. There is no evidence to show that the benefits to using it outweigh the risks. Still, 20–40 percent of all labors that start spontaneously are later augmented.

Even strictly from a physical standpoint, there are numerous natural ways to speed up the progression of labor (although I question if we should even desire to do so). As previously mentioned, walking, nipple stimulation, and baths or showers have all been found to be helpful. However, the most effective means of stimulating labor may actually be engaging in the act of sex. It has been observed that people in tribal cultures often had sex during the early stages of labor. Now there is clinical proof that the hormone relaxin, which softens the cervix and lengthens the pelvic ligaments, is found in seminal plasma. In addition to this, clitoral stimulation and orgasms cause the body to produce oxytocin.

Marilyn Moran writes in her article "The Effect of Lovemaking on the Progress of Labor,"

> Passionate kisses, nipple stimulation (oral as well as manual), perineal massage and support, clitoral stimulation, and coitus early in labor which provides seminal fluid rich in relaxin (the hormone responsible for "extraordinary separation" of the pubic bones as well as softening the cervix) constitute the means for achieving the desired end. . . . Tender warm kisses are especially helpful in getting the mother to relax and allow her body to give birth. (Moran 1993:231–233)

Moran quotes testimony (1993:233–237) to this, as when one woman says, "Lou gave me one of his long Italian kisses. Within seconds that baby door flew open and with one huge contraction . . . the baby descended all the way down the birth canal and his head was ready to emerge." Another woman writes, "This time, for us, what got the baby in also helped to get the baby out. If I hadn't been there myself, and the results hadn't been so instantaneous, I hardly would have believed it."

The hospital environment, however, is not conducive to making love. Therefore, when a woman's labor is not progressing at the "appropriate" speed, Pitocin is often administered.

> Every time I begin to plot a woman's labor curve, I feel that I am signing a death warrant. Sometimes I imagine I'm a guard at a concentration camp, admitting unsuspecting women who, if they do not behave according to the rules, will be sent to the gas chambers. (Harrison 1982:193)

FREQUENT VAGINAL EXAMINATIONS

Almost all pregnant women are subjected to numerous vaginal examinations from the onset of their pregnancy through the delivery of their baby. According to Michel Odent, frequent vaginal examinations are unnecessary and may actually be detrimental. Not only can they lead to vaginal infections, especially if an amniotomy has been done; they can also be quite painful for the laboring woman. Simply observing a woman's body movements, Odent says, and listening to her breathing can tell a doctor or midwife more about the progression of her labor than the insertion of a finger.

Judith Goldsmith lists lack of vaginal examinations in labor as one of the reasons for the overall superiority of tribal births. The frequent checking of dilation, she writes, interferes with a woman's ability to relax.

EPISIOTOMY

An episiotomy is the cutting of the perineum to enlarge the birth opening. It is done supposedly to reduce the risk of tearing and to allow for easier passage of the baby. Approximately 71 percent of all women who give birth in hospitals receive this procedure. Even Robert Bradley, who shows good insight in *Husband-coached Childbirth* (1965) when comparing animal births to human births, believes episiotomies should be done because, after giving birth without one (he says), the vagina will never return to its original shape.

In reality, research has shown that women who have received episiotomies are five to seven times more likely to have a severe laceration than those who have not. This is because, when cut, skin (like cloth) tears much more easily than it would have normally. The cut actually helps initiate the tear. Physician Michelle Harrison writes in *A Woman in Residence* (1982) that she rarely does episiotomies because she finds tears actually heal more quickly and easily than a surgical cut.

In *Birth as an American Rite of Passage* (1992), Robbie Davis-Floyd states that the combination of the episiotomy and the supine position offer the laboring woman the greatest chance of receiving a deep perineal laceration. Besides, they are almost always unnecessary. There are several natural ways of enlarging the birth opening of a woman who is not able on her own to relax sufficiently. Midwives and tribal women have long been aware of the technique of applying hot compresses to a woman's perineum. Massaging olive oil into the skin has also been found to be very effective.

> I had requested no pudendal block or episiotomy, but I got them anyway. Corinth was born at eight pounds, five ounces. They took her away. Every time a needle went into my mutilated perineum, it hurt thanks to the Demerol antidote counteracting the Novocain. It took the episiotomy over a year to stop hurting. I was depressed and humiliated, but it was over. (*Two Attune* 1992, #8:5)

> I was cut through my anal sphincter, through the muscles. I could hardly walk for two months. The haphazard stitches came out two days later. (*New Nativity* 1977, #44:1)

INSTRUMENT DELIVERY

When a baby is not coming out as quickly as a doctor would like, often he will resort to forceps or vacuum extraction. Instrument delivery is employed in approximately 1/3 of all hospital births, with some hospitals going as high as 50 percent. The majority of these are called "elective low forceps." According to the textbook

William's Obstetrics, that means "the obstetrician elects to interfere knowing that it is not absolutely necessary for spontaneous delivery may normally be expected within approximately fifteen minutes" (as told by Korte and Scaer 1990:146).

The necessity of forceps is often precipitated by the use of obstetric drugs, which generally make it more difficult for a woman to push her baby out.

The use of forceps can often result in serious lacerations to the mother's perineum as well as hemorrhaging of the infant's brain and damage to the nerves serving her face and arms. Occasionally, it can even lead to death. In a letter to the newsletter *Two Attune*, one woman wrote,

> After 12 hours of labor . . . the doctor attempted a mid-forceps delivery to rotate the baby into the proper position. This failed due to the cord being wrapped around Mark's chest and neck—loosely, but nevertheless, in a vulnerable position. . . . An emergency section was done and my son was born limp and blue. He was resuscitated but had suffered severe asphyxia due to a lack of oxygen. They believed he compressed the cord—probably while the doctor was trying to turn him with the forceps. He died at 5½ days. . . I can't help but feel Mark may have been safer at home! (*Two Attune* 1992, #6:14)

In another letter to *Two Attune*, a more "fortunate" woman wrote about her baby who was also "assisted" with forceps.

> Our first child was born with her left side paralyzed, her right ear nearly torn off her head, a tear on her right cheek that took three stitches to close, the back of her skull fractured and her clavicle bone fractured. All the doctor had to say was, "It doesn't matter, it's a girl." He was a Navy doctor. There was never once any medical need for any of the interventions he used, other than his convenience and "to speed things up."(*Two Attune* 1991, #4:13)

CESAREAN SECTION

When all else fails, or even when it doesn't, doctors often resort to Cesarean sections. According to an article in *Parade* magazine titled "Are Births as Safe as They Could Be?" (February 7, 1993), the C-section rate in this country is now over 30 percent. With nearly 990,000 C-sections being performed each year, it is the most common major surgery in the United States. According to doctors, these are the reasons C-sections are done:

- because a mother has had a previous C-section
- abnormal labor
- fetal distress
- breech position of baby
- cephalopelvic disproportion

In my mind it is understandable that a labor may be deemed abnormal or a baby may be said to be in distress after undergoing some or all of the many interventions previously listed.

Jane Dwinell, R.N., writes in her book *Birth Stories: Mystery, Power, and Creation* that cephalopelvic disproportion is often a "throw-away excuse from a doctor to describe a baby and a pelvis that didn't seem to fit together" (1992:81). Most likely, Dwinell says, the woman's labor did not conform to the Friedman curve, and the doctor decided he wasn't in the mood to be patient. Dwinell tells the story of a woman whose first baby had been delivered by Cesarean after a diagnosis of cephalopelvic disproportion. When the baby weighed in at nine pounds, the doctor felt his actions had been justified; but the woman wasn't convinced. When she became pregnant with her second baby, she decided she wanted to give birth vaginally in a birthing center. Dwinell witnessed the successful vaginal birth of her 11½ pound son.

Other women tell of similar cases of misdiagnosis that have resulted in unnecessary surgery. Jessica Mitford tells the story of Sharon who went to the hospital after going into labor before her due date. The doctor ordered that a sonogram be done. The sonogram technician reported that the test showed the baby had an abnormal head. Sharon was rushed by ambulance to Sacramento, eighty-five miles away, where her baby was delivered by C-section. One day later Sharon was informed by the doctors that the diagnosis of the sonogram technician had been wrong: the baby was normal. She was then presented with the hospital bill of $11,000, exclusive of the physicians' fee.

Of course, there are numerous factors involved, but much of what is deemed stressful to the infant and mother may be minor compared to the stresses of undergoing a C-section. After a C-section, babies have a higher incidence of jaundice, respiratory distress, high blood pressure, and abnormal neurological responses. Some studies show a mother is at least ten times more likely to die during or after a C-section than she is with a vaginal delivery. One study claimed the rate of maternal deaths associated with Cesareans to be twenty-six times higher. Some women who have undergone C-sections report having a good deal of pain even after several months. Almost half of Cesarean mothers have serious complications from the surgery, including infections, hemorrhaging, sterilization, and injury to other organs.

For doctors, performing a C-section is a lot less time consuming than waiting around for a baby to be born. Mitford cites a study that shows the C-section rate of some doctors soars above 75 percent just before major holidays such as Thanksgiving, Christmas, and New Year's Eve.

Physicians, however, should not have to accept total responsibility for the Cesarean epidemic. Some women also find vaginal birth too time consuming, unpredictable, painful, or simply frightening and actually elect to have a C-section even though they may not be experiencing any physical problems. In Brazil it is quite common for a wealthy woman to opt for a C-section so as not to interfere with her social schedule. This is one reason why the C-section rate in private clinics in Brazil is 90–95 percent.

Cesareans usually cost at least $2,000 more than vaginal deliveries—which leads many people to believe some doctors may have a monetary incentive to perform them. In Brazil, clinics actually encourage women to have C-sections. "Would you like to keep your vagina honeymoon fresh?" is a suggestion made regularly to pregnant Brazilian women (as it appears in Korte and Scaer, 1990). In a *New York Times* article on January 4, 1977, Dr. Paolo Belfort de Aguiar, the former president of the Brazilian Federation of Gynecology and Obstetrics Associations, is quoted as saying, "A substantial number of physicians in Brazil believe that the surgical delivery is the best method of childbirth—it causes no harm to the figure, it is quick, and it is a lot more profitable" (as it appears in Harrison 1982:194). American doctors are not quite so bold, but they reap the benefits just the same.

Some physicians claim that the increase in the percentage of Cesareans performed in this country (from 5 percent of all births in 1970 to 30 percent of all births in 1993) has also led to a lower infant mortality rate. This may be true. However, most European countries have also lowered their infant mortality rates; in fact they're much lower than ours. Still, the percentage of European babies delivered by Cesarean has stayed at 5 percent.

"If I don't section her, the patient might sue me" has become the cry of many physicians when confronted with the abhorrent Cesarean rate. People are suing physicians in record numbers, especially in the field of obstetrics. If a woman is sectioned and a baby is born dead or brain damaged (even though it may have been caused by the Cesarean itself!), the doctor feels he can at least say, "I did everything I could." Even if the fear of lawsuits were an acceptable excuse for doing unnecessary surgery, it's still merely a superficial, Band-Aid solution to a multifaceted problem.

> I was diagnosed as "failure to progress." I tell people it was failure to be patient on their part. The baby was fine. There was never any fetal distress. I felt like I got ripped off here. A lot of grieving was involved. Sadness. Because it was something that was so important, so emotional. More than anything I wanted to hold my baby in my arms immediately after birth. And here because of technology and impatience, I missed that. Your God-given ability to birth your baby is taken away. (Abbott 1992a)

> The woman today had a fine uterus, but we have rules that say she can only give birth in a certain way and she did not follow our rules, so we cut open her belly. But we cut in the wrong place and now she will probably never have kids again. Now she will probably have problems with intercourse. We have really ripped apart her insides and sewn them back together again, but they are not the way they were. The woman was so close to delivering and the baby's head was so far down that he had to have someone go under the

drapes to push the baby's head back up into her uterus. (Harrison 1982:167)

SUCTIONING OF THE BABY'S NOSE AND MOUTH AFTER BIRTH

Almost all babies are routinely suctioned immediately after birth. Overproduction of the mucous membranes only occurs when a baby is under considerable stress; so, for many babies, there is no mucus there to be suctioned out. Generally the doctor does it anyway—"just in case."

Mucus catheters, however, may not only be unnecessary; they may be dangerous as well. Sheila Kitzinger quotes Dr. Donald Garrow's testimony to this in her book *Birth at Home:* "Sticking a catheter down a baby's throat is bad. Pushing it into a baby's mouth and nose does nothing at all to help it breathe. Mucus catheters should be banned as dangerous instruments" (1979:40).

Kitzinger writes that, if a baby has some excess mucus after birth, she should be held or placed on her tummy with her head slightly lower than her body. This will allow the mucus to drain out on its own. Often a baby may sneeze and clear out her airways without assistance.

EARLY CLAMPING OF THE CORD AND INSISTENCE ON IMMEDIATE DETACHMENT OF THE PLACENTA

It is common practice in most hospitals to clamp the umbilical cord immediately after birth. According to Dr. William F. Windle writing in *Scientific American*, this can be dangerous.

To clamp the cord immediately is equivalent to subjecting the infant to a massive hemorrhage, because almost a fourth of the fetal blood is in the placental circuit at birth. Depriving the infant of that much blood can be a factor in exacerbating an incipient hypoxemia and can thus contribute to the danger of asphyxial brain damage. (Windle 1969:77)

Marion Sousa, author of *Childbirth at Home* (1976), states that early clamping of the cord can lead to hemorrhaging in the mother and retention of the placenta. She advises birth attendants to refrain from clamping the cord until after it has turned white and stopped pulsating.

In most hospital deliveries, a woman is expected to expel the placenta within five to ten minutes after giving birth. This is simply an arbitrary time limit imposed by physicians. Couples who have given birth at home, without medical assistance, report it is not uncommon for a placenta to take as long as two to three hours to detach. One woman wrote in the newsletter *The New Nativity* that she had delivered a fully intact, healthy placenta fourteen hours after giving birth.

However, since most home-birth babies are nursed immediately after birth, generally the placenta is not long in coming. When a woman is not permitted to nurse her baby within the first few minutes, often the placenta does not detach because there is a lack of sufficient oxytocin in her system. Pitocin, therefore, is often "required" to assist its release.

VITAMIN K AND EYE DROPS

Almost all babies in hospitals are given a shot of vitamin K immediately after birth, supposedly because babies are born "deficient." Simply allowing a baby to nurse after birth will alleviate this problem. The colostrum in a woman's breasts is rich in vitamin K.

Silver nitrate, or something comparable, is put in most babies' eyes, supposedly to prevent blindness should the mother have gonorrhea. A simple test on the mother before the birth, if she so desires, would seem kinder to the infant. Any solution put into the eyes at birth is considerably irritating. It also interferes with the baby's ability to see for several days. Occasionally an infant has been blinded by the administering of too much silver nitrate by an incompetent intern.

SEPARATION OF THE MOTHER AND BABY
AFTER BIRTH

Although "rooming in" has become more common in recent years, many babies are still taken to the nursery after birth, supposedly to allow the mother to recuperate and to protect the baby from possible "germs." Earl Ubell writes in his article "Are Births as Safe as They Could Be?"

> Evidence shows that generally it is much safer for the infants to room with their mothers, in whose bodies, after all, they were carried and nurtured, and very likely instilled with immunities. In the nursery, on the other hand, germs spread to the healthy infants from the sick ones. (Ubell 1993:10)

From a psychological standpoint, separating the mother and baby can be emotionally devastating for both of them. Although many people scoff at the concept of bonding, there is a significant amount of research to prove that the first several hours of a child's life should most definitely be spent in the arms of it's mother or father.

In a ten-year study conducted at Oxford University in England, it was found that babies who were separated from their mothers after birth—even for so short a time as four hours—were more apt to be abused by their mothers in later years. Of course, it doesn't take a scientific study to convince most mothers that separating them from their babies after birth is harmful. It's simply common sense.

I will admit that, in rare cases, intervention is a necessary evil and thankfully there are skilled physicians who can help save the life of a mother or baby. However, as I have stated, intervening in birth is not rare. It is routine.

Many mothers object to intervention but find they are forced, or forcibly coerced, into receiving it when they put themselves into a hospital environment. In a letter to Anthony M. Ludivici in *The Truth about Childbirth* a woman wrote,

> In my own case I had some difficulty in deciding if I was in labour as I experienced no pain at all but only a periodic feeling of distension, similar to a distension of the bowel. . . . It was fun, breathless and exciting like bathing in a rough sea. Then someone put a mask over my face. I pushed it off and told them I didn't want it. They took no notice and I had to let them have their way. (Ludivici 1938:v)

In his book *Childbirth without Fear*, Grantly Dick-Read relayed the following birth experience:

> I felt the baby would be born quickly and easily. I was ordered to take gas by the sisters. "I don't want any," I said. The nurse tried to force me to take ether. I was resentful and indignant. I was even slapped for not taking gas when I bore down. (Dick-Read 1959:175)

For those who would argue that times have changed, let me cite Diana Korte and Roberta Scaer, authors of *A Good Birth, A Safe Birth* (1990), who—more than thirty years after *Childbirth without Fear* was written—asked women about their experiences in birth. One woman wrote,

> Because of my last experience, I am convinced that the majority of gyn doctors are not the least bit interested in the mother's preferences in childbirth. They seek the safest and quickest way to immobilize you and pull your baby out, regardless of your insistence that you are experiencing no discomfort and wish to have no drugs. I was not permitted to labor and deliver in the same bed, to have my hands free, or to nurse my child immediately following delivery. There was no medical reason for denying me these things, especially after we had talked about these very points before my delivery, and the doctors had all agreed. My doctor was able to harass me into having a spinal, which was being administered under my protests as my new son slipped into the world. I was in the hospital exactly forty-two minutes before my child was born, and it was filled with tears and loud arguing between my doctors and myself. Thank God it was not my first pregnancy, for if it were, I would surely not have another. (Korte and Scaer 1990:24–25)

Unfortunately, these are not isolated incidences. In an article in the *Sunday Times* (London, June 13, 1982), a woman was quoted as saying,

They tried to give me drugs, and I and my mother who was with me, said I absolutely didn't want anything. Then the nurse called the sister, who arrived with an injection of 100 milligrams of pethidine, and against my will, simply stuck it into me. (as it appeared in *New Nativity* 1987, #41:7)

To add insult to injury, this same woman was arrested several years later for giving birth to a healthy baby at home without medical assistance. Unlike in the United States where, for the most part, unassisted birth is permitted, it is illegal in England.

Of course, not all hospital births are horrendous. Many women are treated well in hospitals. Their wishes are respected. They have supportive birth attendants and are allowed to give birth in the way they desire.

Often, however, a woman who speaks glowingly about her physician and the interventions that he deemed necessary may not be facing up to the reality of the situation. According to one childbirth educator I spoke with, many women develop a "hostage" mentality when in the hospital. As with hostages, they actually begin to identify with their "captors." They may say, "Everyone was so nice to me. Yes, I had a Cesarean, but my doctor said that when a baby is over eight pounds a woman almost always has to be sectioned." Many women simply feel more comfortable rationalizing their experiences than analyzing them and possibly coming to the conclusion that they and their trusted physicians did something wrong.

Occasionally a doctor is so adamant in his desire to intervene in a birth that he resorts to using the legal system to enforce his decision. In 1986, a national survey revealed there had been twenty-one attempts to obtain court orders to force pregnant women to receive obstetrical intervention. Fifteen of these were for Cesarean sections. In Beth Shearer's article "Forced Cesareans: The Case of the Disappearing Mothers," she gives the following example:

In a 1981 Georgia case, doctors told the court there was a 99 percent chance of fetal death and a 50 percent chance of maternal death unless a scheduled Cesarean section was performed, since two ultrasounds indicated a complete placenta praevia (a potentially life-threatening situation in which the placenta lies under the baby, blocking the entrance to the birth canal). The mother steadfastly believed in her ability to give birth safely. After the court order was granted, a third ultrasound showed no praevia at all. (Shearer 1989:7)

In 1982 a judge and an attorney were summoned to a Denver hospital room where a woman was refusing to have a Cesarean. The doctor believed the baby was in distress, so the judge declared it a ward of the state until after its birth. The woman was forcibly anesthetized and a Cesarean was performed. The baby was born perfectly healthy.

Many doctors insist that birth is inherently dangerous and therefore their actions are justified. Many people, including some physicians, are beginning to question that premise.

Dr. Henry Jellett, former master of the Rotunda Hospital in Dublin, Ireland, believes the maternal mortality rate would be much lower if women were left unaided in childbirth. "Is there a single incident in the management of normal labour which is not opposed to the physiological process of labour?" (as quoted in Ludivici 1938:21). Dr. B. F. Macchia concurs. "Nature," he says, "is not having much of a chance" (as quoted in Ludivici 1938:21).

Perhaps the greatest gift the modern-day physician can offer a woman is that of his absence at the time of birth.

Chapter Three

The Psychological Effects of a Traumatic Birth on a Family

Imagine a primal psychology which includes the imprint, for both men and women, of co-creating tremendous, somatic pleasure during birth. The implications for a template of sexuality based on ecstasy, rather than extreme pain, are provocative. Would we see less sado-masochistic behavior in sexuality? Would rape decrease if men and women felt less like the cause, or at least an involuntary accomplice of suffering at birth?

—Jeannine Parvati Baker

As I have shown in Chapter 2, when a woman buys into the technocratic model of birth, both physically and psychologically, often she ends up hurting both herself and her baby. Forceps, drugs, Cesareans, and other interventions sometimes maim a child for life. Unseen, however, is the psychological devastation incurred not only by the child, but by the mother and father as well.

THE CHILD

In the field of psychology, it is an almost universally accepted fact that birth trauma is a source of many of our emotional problems. Author Otto Rank claims, however, that all illness, both physical and mental, can be traced back to the trauma of birth. Often, he says, a child who has undergone a traumatic birth will never again trust her mother or the physical universe. In *The Trauma of Birth* Rank writes, "We shall take as our guiding principle Freud's statement that all anxiety goes back originally to the anxiety at birth. . . . [E]very infantile utterance of anxiety or fear is really a partial disposal of the birth anxiety" (1952:11–17).

Migraines, he says, are a remembrance of the pressure felt on the head in a difficult birth. Asthma is an attempt by the frightened child to return to the prebirth environment where breathing was unnecessary. Gerald Heard agrees. In *The Five Ages of Man* he writes,

> The child strives not to grow but to return to the womb. . . . [The] frightened infant, instead of breathing, may actually go back to womb lung reflexes, refusing to fill the lung with air and forcing the emptied lung down on the diaphragm. This is the reflex whereby in the prenatal state, the fetus helped to draw in more oxygenated blood through the umbilical cord, but which now in the postnatal state can only result in suffocation. (Heard 1963:100–101)

Many physicians who have worked with asthmatic children have commented that the seizures seem to be brought on by specific emotional situations that often involve the mother. In *Psychic Phenomena* (1967) Robert Bradley tells the story of an asthmatic boy who only had breathing difficulties when he was around his mother. Another asthmatic child would have an attack simply if it was mentioned that his mother was coming to visit.

The fact that the mother may have been drugged at birth and didn't herself necessarily (or consciously) view the experience as traumatic doesn't mean the child was unaffected. To the contrary, say some psychologists, the drugs actually add to the trauma of birth.

Some physicians mistakenly argue that obstetric drugs given to a woman in labor make for a more satisfying psychological experience for the mother, and that therefore the baby must benefit as well. Many women agree. A woman once said to me, "The epidural relaxed me so much that I ended up enjoying the birth. Otherwise

I wouldn't have. Isn't that better for both me and my baby, at least from a psychological standpoint, than enduring a nightmare of pain?"

One's first response might be yes. However, studies show that babies who have been subjected to obstetric drugs at birth have a higher rate of chemical dependency as adults. This, says Robbie Davis-Floyd in *Birth as an American Rite of Passage* (1992), is not due so much to physical factors as it is to psychological ones. The child has been taught from the moment of her birth that drugs are the best way to deal with problems and pain in life.

In a study (1987) conducted by Dr. Bertil Jacobson and his colleagues at Sweden's Karolinska Institute, it was found that a child may actually be imprinted at birth in the same way that baby birds are. A chick becomes emotionally and physically attached to the first thing it sees after birth. Jacobson believes human babies also become imprinted at birth, but all too often the first things they encounter during and immediately after birth are obstetric drugs, various machines and instruments, and hospital personnel. This unnatural dependency developed at birth may continue throughout the child's life.

Jacobson carried out case-controlled studies of 412 suicide victims and drug addicts in Stockholm. He and his colleagues concluded that

> suicide involving asphyxiation was associated with asphyxiation at birth, suicide by violent mechanical means was associated with mechanical birth trauma, and drug addiction was associated with opiate and/or barbiturate administration to mothers during labor. [This suggests that the mechanism transferring birth trauma to adulthood is] analogous to imprinting in animals. (Jacobson et al. 1987:364)

Babies grow up to give birth to their own babies, but their memories stay with them. Psychotherapist Gayle Peterson believes women carry their own traumatic experiences in birth with them into adulthood, adversely affecting their labors. In *Birthing Normally* she writes, "Many of the complications of birth experienced by women today may have an association to their own alienation in birth. . . . [That is why] it can prove very helpful to an individual woman to explore the experience of her own birth" (1981:165).

If a woman realizes her birth was traumatic, she can then take steps to change it through various rebirthing exercises. (Peterson points out that birth itself is not traumatic. However, the techno-cratic birth—with its numerous medical procedures and accompanying expectations of disaster—is.)

In the past twenty years, the concept of rebirthing has become very popular. But according to Gerald Heard in *The Five Ages of Man* (1963), rebirthing ceremonies have been occurring for centuries. Baptism, he claims, was originally designed as a rebirthing exercise. (It has since become a supposed ritual of purification, reinforcing the belief that individuals are "impure" without official sanction.)

People who have studied rebirthing believe that memories of birth, once confronted, may be psychologically altered. When a person decides to be rebirthed, generally she (or he) is placed in a large tub of water to simulate the prebirth environment. A rebirth-ing practitioner then leads her through a series of exercises that help her to remember her own birth. After releasing her previously repressed emotions, she is told to create imaginatively the type of birth she would have liked to experience.

Often, women who have been through the rebirthing process claim it helped them in their own labors. Here again, I have no doubt that it did; however, I believe we are perfectly capable of rebirthing ourselves. We need only to relax and imagine vividly the birth we would have liked to have. We don't necessary need to dwell on the unpleasant aspects of our own birth, nor do we need to hide from them. The emphasis should be on our desires, how-ever.

Another undesirable consequence of a traumatic birth, as Jean-nine Parvati Baker alluded to in the quote at the beginning of this chapter, is the guilt a child feels when she undoubtedly blames herself for her mother's ordeal. Sometimes a mother tells the child directly how much she suffered in order to bring her into the world. More often than not, however, the mother herself is unaware of the feelings of resentment she has toward her child. Either that, or she chooses not to express them. Still, the feelings are there, and they affect the child in numerous ways.

THE MOTHER

After a traumatic birth, a woman is likely to feel frightened, frustrated, and inadequate. Postpartum depression—a condition that my generation was told is a natural part of the birth process—only occurs, claims author Helen Wessel, after an unnatural, medically controlled birth. In *Natural Childbirth and the Christian Family* she writes,

> The most important contributing factor to depression following childbirth is a feeling of being robbed, a sense of loss. For nine months of pregnancy and several hours of labor, a woman has been gradually brought to a peak of emotional and physical expectation. An adequate emotional and physical climax at the moment of birth provides a most essential catharsis for this pent-up emotion. This climax is essential. A mother who has missed it and had a passive, frigid birth, due to anesthetics . . . still is emotionally in a state of expectancy. She looks at her child, but experiences no euphoria, no sense of exhilaration. . . . If an adequate birth climax does not provide it, it will come later, in spells of frustrated weeping, like the tantrums of frustration of the small child who cannot explain, and indeed does not know, what it is he wants. (Wessel 1963:209–210)

Psychiatrist James Clark Moloney says he doesn't even like to use the term "postpartum depression" because it infers a physiological basis.

> I want, first and foremost, to rob the cliché of the so-called "third-day depression" of any element of physiological consistency. There is no physiological responsibility behind a mental depression. A mental depression is a psychological manifestation and it is a complete trend of events that takes place as a result of frustration. (quoted in Wessel 1963:209)

Many mothers speak of feeling that they have somehow failed after undergoing a difficult birth, especially if it resulted in a Cesarean. The fact that the baby is often taken to a nursery (to allow the mother to recuperate) greatly adds to her sense of loneliness, guilt, and frustration. One Cesarean mother wrote, "After the birth I felt miserable, agonizingly miserable . . . and ashamed. I felt so ashamed of myself for screaming, and for not being able to do it" (as quoted in Davis-Floyd 1992:233). Another woman wrote, "I cannot live with the thought of my birth experience. It gives me the shudders, and I start to cry every time I think about it. So I don't think about it. It's over and done, and life goes on" (as quoted in Davis-Floyd 1992:242).

Unfortunately, an unpleasant experience doesn't end simply because it is no longer physically occurring. The fear, shame, and guilt associated with a traumatic birth creeps into every aspect of a woman's life. Her sexual and emotional relationship with her husband may never again be the same. Fear of another pregnancy or unpleasant memories of the first one may interfere with her ability to be intimate.

On the *Sally Jessy Raphael Show* (March 10, 1993), a woman stated that, every time she and her husband began to have sex, neither one of them could get rid of the image of her lying on a table with her belly sliced open and EKG jelly on her breasts.

Other women have stated that, although it may not be justified, often they blame their husbands for the pain and humiliation they endured during birth. In a letter to *Two Attune* a woman wrote,

> The hospital births left me feeling extremely depressed and I'd bawl all the time and would almost feel hatred toward the doctor and the others in the hospital whom I felt were just plain abusive. I did not feel close with my husband after those births either; in fact, I was angry with him for allowing them to do all the things they did to me. The last time we were there I told him later on, "How can you stand to even watch them doing all that crap to me?" I told him it might sound weird to him, but I felt like I was practically being raped and that he just stood by and watched and allowed it. (*Two Attune* 1991, #4:14)

THE FATHER

Even if a woman doesn't blame her husband for the problems she encountered in birthing, he may still blame himself. Guilt in our society is directed so intensely toward men, regarding the suffering that women "must" endure, that many men are reluctant to become fathers at all. One man told me, "I desperately want to have children but I don't want to put my wife through all that pain."

Men who have witnessed their wives enduring a difficult birth often report they are unable to rid themselves of the belief that they were responsible or at least a party to their wife's pain. Robert Bradley tells of a conversation he had with a father who was reluctant to accompany his wife into the delivery room for the birth of their third child. After much encouragement the man still refused, stating,

> Doc, I sat out in that waiting room for hours with the other two. I could hear her screaming through two sets of closed doors, and they told me they were giving her all the medicine they dared. Doc, I get sick to my stomach when I hear her scream and realize I got her pregnant. (quoted in Bradley 1965:63)

No doubt more than a few marriages have degenerated after the birth of a baby at least in part due to the circumstances of its birth.

Until we consciously decide as individuals to free ourselves from the technocratic model of birth, this cycle of pain and misery is bound to continue.

Chapter Four

Why Physicians Insist on Intervening

You have to consider—and beware of—the doctor's self interest. Doctors almost always get more reward and recognition
for *intervening* than for not intervening. They're trained to
intervene and do something rather than observe, wait, and
take the chance the patient will get better all by himself or go
to another doctor. As a matter of fact, one of my key pieces
of subversive advice to medical students is this: To pass an
exam, get through medical school, and retain your sanity,
always choose the most interventionist answer on a multiple
choice test and you're likely to be right. . . . This piece of
advice has carried more of my students through various cru-
cial examinations, including national boards and specialty
exams, than any other lesson.

—Robert S. Mendelsohn, M.D.,
Confessions of a Medical Heretic

Ask almost any physician why a baby should be born in the
hospital, given the extent of unnecessary and often dangerous
intervention, and he will tell you, "It's better than the alternative."
Better for whom?

Numerous studies have been conducted over the past twenty
years that show not only is home birth just as safe as hospital birth,
but often it has been found to be safer.

Perhaps the best known study was conducted in 1977 by Lewis Mehl, M.D. (as reported in Davis-Floyd 1992:179) Mehl did a comparative study of 1,046 planned home births and 1,046 planned hospital births. After the births were analyzed for length of labor, complications, outcomes for the infants, and procedures utilized, he found that home birth was actually safer than hospital birth for both the mother and the baby.

The hospital births had a five times higher incidence of maternal high blood pressure, three and a half times more meconium staining (indicative of fetal distress), eight times more shoulder dystocia (due in part to the insistence on the supine position for delivery), and three times the rate of postpartum hemorrhage (primarily due to early clamping of the cord and attempts made to remove a placenta manually before it was ready to come out). Three times as many hospital babies required resuscitation (primarily due to medication), and four times as many became infected. Thirty times as many hospital babies suffered birth injuries (due to forceps). The injuries consisted of severe cephalhematoma (a collection of blood beneath the scalp), fractured skull, fractured clavicle, facial nerve paralysis, brachial nerve injury, eye injury, and so on.

Less than 5 percent of the home-birth mothers received analgesia or anesthesia, compared to more than 75 percent of the women in hospitals. C-sections were three times more frequent in the hospital group than in the planned home group. Women in the hospital had nine times as many episiotomies and nine times as many severe tears. Both the maternal and neonatal death rates were the same for both groups.

Other studies have had similar results, and some even show the rate for maternal and neonatal deaths to be greater in hospitals. English research statistician, Marjorie Tew conducted a study during the 1970s and 1980s comparing home birth, and births taking place in freestanding birth centers, to hospital birth. The 16,328 births she evaluated were classified into risk categories of very low, low, moderate, high, and very high. In *every* category the neonatal mortality rate was lower *out* of the hospital. At the very low and low levels of risk, two to three times as many babies died in the hospital. At the moderate level, eight times as many; and at the high level, three times as many babies died in the hospital. Tew concluded that care by obstetricians is not only incapable, save in exceptional cases, of reducing predicted risk . . . it actually provokes and adds to the dangers . . . [T]he emotional security of a familiar setting, the home, makes a greater contribution to safety than does the equipment in hospital to facilitate obstetric interventions in cases of emergency. (Tew 1990:267)

In a study done between 1960 and 1969 in Newcastle upon Tyne, a town in England, it was found that more babies died in hospital deliveries than in home deliveries. In 1986 the perinatal mortality rate in Dutch hospitals was 13.9 per thousand, compared to 2.2 per thousand for home births. Robbie Davis-Floyd (1992) writes that studies done in Arizona, Canada, and Tennessee demonstrate the relative safety and viability of home birth.

Sheila Kitzinger agrees. In *Birth at Home* she writes,

One of the reasons why some women want to give birth at home is that many hospitals are not good enough. They are not good enough to provide an environment suited for a peak experience of one's life, nor for the birth of a family. But more than this, they are sometimes frankly dangerous places in which to have a baby. (Kitzinger 1979:5)

Why then do doctors insist that babies be born in hospitals? Why do they insist that medical intervention is necessary in spite of mounting evidence that shows it is not?

One obvious answer is ignorance. Many doctors are caring individuals who are simply unaware of the fact that what they're doing is dangerous. "Women are nailed upon the Cross of Pain [in childbirth]," writes Pat Carter, "only because their would be benefactors do not know what harm they do" (1957:46). Doctors have been taught that birth is a pathological condition requiring their assistance; and in all honesty, they believe they are genuinely helping humanity. However, as they say, the road to hell is paved with good intentions.

Obstetrician John Franklin shares Robert Mendelsohn's belief that doctors are simply doing what they've been trained to do.

> Every doctor enjoys his intervention. That's what his skill and
> training are for. Some think that nature is in constant need of
> improvement and others that nature can't be trusted, but one
> kind of intervention leads to another and then the doctor is
> kept busy seeking remedies for his own actions. (Franklin,
> quoted in Korte and Scaer 1990:109)

Of course, another obvious answer to the question of intervention is money. Childbirth today is a very profitable business ($15
billion annually, to be exact), not only for physicians but for the
pharmaceutical industry as well. Pat Carter tells the story of attempting to buy birthing supplies from the local pharmacist. When
he realized it was for an unassisted home birth, he refused to sell
them to her. Carter writes, "It seems the Medicine has all the
auxiliary sciences—laboratory, pharmaceutical, and what have
you—lined up to protect its 'royalty' rights to the PELVIC GOLD-
MINE. (Women have only squatters rights to their insides.)"
(1957:46).

More than money is involved, however. Physician Michelle
Harrison says it has to do with control. In *A Woman in Residence*
(1982), Harrison writes about coming across an article that showed
the benefits of allowing a woman to walk while in labor. Initially
she thought her colleagues would be interested, but then she
realized their insistence on bed rest for laboring women was not
based on their desire to aid as much as it was to control. She
suddenly saw physicians *insisting* that women walk while in labor,
because "they" had now determined it was the thing to do.

Doctors are no different from the rest of society. In every field
there are people who have unresolved emotional and psychological problems. Often they are all too willing to ignore their own
feelings of inadequacy and instead attempt to dominate and control others. We can see it in political leaders and religious zealots;
but somehow, when it occurs in the medical field, it is socially
acceptable because physicians are supposedly intelligent, enlight-
ened individuals who certainly must know what's best for us.

The following quote from a fourth-year resident shows the
desire many physicians have to be the "leader of the band."

Well, I sort of see my role at birth this way: I am the captain of the team, and the mother and the father and the nurses—they are all players. If somebody is going to call the shots, it's going to be me. Sometimes the mother calls the shots, but mostly it's me. (quoted in Davis-Floyd 1992:268)

Perhaps many doctors have misplaced technical skills and would be better off working with machines. The little boy in a poor family who enjoys taking things apart may be encouraged to pursue a career in mechanics, whereas the wealthy one, or one with wealthy inclinations, may be encouraged to go into medicine. Women, however, are not machines and they are not designed to be taken apart. A person who enjoys doing this either has valuable technical skills that should be used on machines and not on people, or else has masochistic tendencies and should not be allowed to work in obstetrics and gynecology.

To the truly dedicated ob/gyns I say, "Thank you, and please ignore this chapter." Unfortunately there are too many doctors who, upon close examination, cannot be considered to be truly dedicated.

Dr. Rhoda Nussbaum, head of obstetrics at Kaiser Permanente in San Francisco, believes that many a physician who works with women does not have their best interests in mind.

My impression of gynecologists as a woman going to one in my teen-age years and early twenties, and later my encounters with them in medical school, is that there were an awful lot of gynecologists who were misogynists, who seemed to have chosen that field as a way to act out their dislike for women. I believe that's true. It's a sweeping generalization, but that was my experience. (quoted in Mitford 1992:103)

Michelle Harrison agrees. "The medical birth is pornographic. The woman is degraded. . . . All day long I watch women who have been violated and who don't even know it" (1982:111).

When Harrison confronted a doctor about the way he had been treating a woman who was giving birth ("Push you lazy female! Push!"), he stated, "Michelle, when people are in a subservient position, sometimes you just have to tell them what to do" (quoted in Harrison 1982:198–199).

According to Melvin Konner, M.D., Ph.D., author of *Becoming a Doctor: A Journey of Initiation in Medical School*, physicians in general may often have a strong dislike of people: "To cut and puncture a person, to take his or her life in your hands, to pound the chest until the ribs break . . . these and a thousand other things may require something stronger than objectivity. They may actually require a measure of dislike" (1987:373).

Robbie Davis-Floyd claims it goes much deeper than simply disliking people.

[Physicians intervene to prove] the necessity for cultural control of natural processes, the untrustworthiness of nature and the associated weakness and inferiority of the female body. . . . [Also,] the validity of patriarchy, the superiority of science and technology, and the importance of institutions and machines. (Davis-Floyd 1993:71)

"Safety" is the disguise worn by technocratic ideology. The real issue in the home versus hospital debate is not safety but the conflict between radically opposed systems of value and belief. (Davis-Floyd 1992:184)

The doctor, in defending his position concerning medical intervention, is actually defending a whole belief system—a system that says, "There is no God or spiritual reality. Whatever nature has produced is inferior to what the official technologically based establishment has produced. Nature is ignorant; technology is supreme. And even if God does exist, with all my years of training I'm smarter than He is!"

In an article in the *St. Louis Globe Democrat* titled "Some Women Prefer Home Births" (Krauska 1976), physician Roy Boedeker spoke of performing an episiotomy. His statement shows the attitude many physicians have concerning the alleged superiority of modern medical techniques: "We inject a little Novocain, make a little cut, lift the baby out gently with forceps, then repair and restore the pelvic floor even better than God made it."

In the newsletter *Two Attune*, a woman described a telling encounter she had with a doctor. After she informed him she wasn't
going to have her labor induced because she chose to wait on God,
the doctor seemed outraged. He told her *he* was the one who had
been to medical school, and walked out without allowing her
another word.

Gerald Heard would describe this arrogant attitude as typical
of what in *The Five Ages of Man* (1963), he calls the "humanic mind."
Believing in materialism (there is no God or spiritual reality—life
just "appeared") is simply one stage that humankind goes through
on its evolutionary path. The so-called scientists of today believe
they have reached the epitome of rational thought, when in reality
they are lost in the woods. The humanic man and woman, however,
do not see their beliefs as merely a temporary step on the way to
enlightenment. They see them as truths, and all too often they are
more than willing to inflict them on the rest of the "uneducated,
ignorant" masses.

"Have your 'faith' if you must," the physician may say, "but I
will be here with my pain killers and surgical instruments when
that fails." Of course, if *that* fails, that says nothing at all about the
inferiority of technocracy.

Perhaps, however, the physician knows—somewhere within
him—that he is not so smart. Perhaps he is aware of something
beyond his physical senses; but because he hasn't taken the time
to explore it, he fears it and anyone who chooses to trust it. "Trust
me," he says, "I have all the answers." But maybe, in reality, he
doesn't trust himself. Maybe he doesn't want to play God anymore.
Are we really doing the medical profession a favor when we say,
"I am nothing. You know best. Take care of me?"

Penny Armstrong, C.N.M., wrote in *A Wise Birth* about her
feelings when dealing with psychologically passive women:

> Sometimes I hated the birthing women for being powerless.
> Sometimes I wanted to shake them, yell at them, insist that
> they stand up for themselves. But then I'd feel the pull of an
> undertow; I'd feel them wanting us to abuse them: I'd feel
> them pleading for the repetition of the pattern in their lives.
> My fury would die. I'd realize that I'd been angry with them
> because they didn't want my respect. (Armstrong 1990:117)

Michelle Harrison echoes Armstrong's sentiments:

> Often I don't like the women I've delivered. I don't like them
> for their submissiveness. . . . For me, the submissiveness of
> one woman becomes my own, as though we were all one
> organism. Their imprisonment adds to my own sense of
> powerlessness in this hospital. (Harrison 1982:129)

Although both Harrison and Armstrong would like to see
women stand up for themselves, I'm sure neither of them would
approve of the degree of autonomy and self-reliance that I am
proposing. They are not quite to the point of wanting to put
themselves out of a job.

This brings to mind a conversation that took place between
Hawkeye Pierce and Colonel Potter on the television series
M*A*S*H. After witnessing the amazing recovery of numerous
patients who had only been given sugar water, Colonel Potter
pointed to his head and said, "You know, the best doctor's right up
here." Hawkeye replied, "Shhh. Don't tell anyone. We'll all be out
of jobs."

Putting oneself out of a job, however, is what physician Robert
Mendelsohn claims should be every doctor's goal. In *Confessions of
a Medical Heretic*, he writes about his vision of the future, and of the
physician whom he calls the "New Doctor":

> Never forget that the New Doctor's goal is to work himself
> or herself right out of business, so your dependence on the
> professional should diminish every day. You have to learn to
> get along without doctors, because doctors aren't the Oracles
> of faith. The Oracles of faith, the true celebrants of the religion
> of life are the *self*, the *family*, and the *community*. From these
> vessels flow the determinants of health: life, love, and cour-
> age. (Mendelsohn 1979:160)

If we are to succeed in childbirth, we must stop viewing physicians, or even midwives, as our saviors. They are human beings—
no more, no less. We are our own saviors. Isn't it time to exercise
our courage and take our lives into our own hands?

Breaking what may have been a lifelong dependence on author-ity figures may take some doing. However, as English writer and philosopher James Allen so eloquently wrote, our efforts will be rewarded with the greatest of all gifts: freedom.

It has been usual for men to think and to say, "Many men are slaves because one is an oppressor; let us hate the oppressor." Now, however, there is among an increasing few a tendency to reverse this judgement, and to say, "One man is an oppres-sor because many are slaves; let us despise the slaves." The truth is that oppressor and slave are cooperators in ignorance, and, while seeming to afflict each other, are in reality afflicting themselves. A perfect Knowledge perceives the action of law in the weakness of the oppressed and the misapplied power of the oppressor. A perfect Love, seeing the suffering which both states entail, condemns neither. A perfect Compassion embraces both oppressor and oppressed. He who has con-quered weakness, and has put away all selfish thoughts, belongs neither to oppressor nor oppressed. He is free. (Allen 1993:46–47)

Chapter Five

Personal Beliefs and Expectations

> You are in physical existence to learn and understand that your energy translated into feelings, thoughts and emotions, causes *all* experience. *There are no exceptions.*
> —Seth/Jane Roberts
> *The Nature of Personal Reality*

As most women who have given birth at home can attest, simply removing oneself from the medical environment does not ensure that a woman will have a painless easy birth. This is because unnecessary medical intervention is only one of the reasons why most Western women have painful, difficult labors.

I mentioned in Chapter 1 that tribal women, because of their level of self-consciousness, have not developed beliefs in fear, shame, and guilt. In order to understand the significance of this in relation to childbirth, we must deal with the concept of belief itself.

Very few people have written as extensively about the power of belief as the late Jane Roberts has. Roberts was a poet and author when, in 1964, she found herself experiencing alterations in her consciousness. Shortly thereafter, she began lapsing into trances, and speaking for an "energy personality essence" who called himself Seth.

At first, both Roberts and her husband were skeptical. The quality of the information given in the sessions was so outstanding, however, that Roberts did not attempt to negate her experiences. Over the course of the next twenty years, Seth dictated more than 6,000 pages of typewritten material (which is now permanently housed in the Yale University Library), dealing with such concepts as the nature of time, dreams, probable realities, physics, and, most importantly, the power of the individual self-conscious personality.

Numerous psychologists had lengthy conversations with Seth over the years, and very few of them doubted his authenticity. Eugene Barnard of North Carolina State University wrote after engaging in a long philosophical discussion with Seth,

> The best summary description I can give you of that evening is that it was for me a delightful conversation with a personality or intelligence or what have you, whose wit, intellect, and reservoir of knowledge far exceeded my own. . . . In any sense in which a psychologist of the Western scientific tradition would understand the phrase, I do not believe that Jane Roberts and Seth are the same person, or the same personality, or different facets of the same personality. (Barnard, as quoted in Talbot 1988:207)

Michael Talbot (author of the popular book *Mysticism and the New Physics*) writes in *Beyond the Quantum,*

> Regardless of the ultimate nature of the Seth phenomenon (a communication from a being no longer focused in physical reality or a product of Robert's unconscious mind), the mere magnitude, coherence, and intellectual quality of what Seth had to say indicate that he was a phenomenon deserving of further scientific study. (Talbot 1988:207)

Writer Raymond Van Over said of the Seth material,

> The best trance material shows good psychological insight communicated through a compassionate, strong personality; and the Seth material conveys all of these qualities. Seth, however, adds one ingredient that most trance material lacks:

clarity of thought and presentation. Most trance material, from ancient as well as modern mediumistic controls, couches itself not only in jumbled syntax but confused thought; however, Seth, I believe, has a great talent for introducing complex and often difficult subjects simply and clearly. (Van Over, in Roberts 1970:xiv)

Seth teaches that we create our own reality according to our desires, beliefs, and intentions. Thoughts, he says, are not merely nebulous words floating about in our heads. They are actually electromagnetic particles, which, once conceived, have an intense desire to manifest themselves in the physical world. The stronger the thought, the more quickly it will come into our experience. In *The Nature of Personal Reality*, Seth says,

The living picture of the world grows within the mind. The world as it appears to you is like a three-dimensional painting in which each individual takes a hand. Each color, each line that appears within it has first been painted within a mind and only then does it materialize without.

In this case, however, the artists themselves are a portion of the painting and appear within it. There is no effect in the exterior world that does not spring from an inner source. There is no motion that does not first occur within the mind. (Roberts 1974:3)

Seth does not say "except" or "but." He says everything that happens to us is the result of our beliefs, from stubbing a toe to dying in a car accident. We may believe that certainly we did not want to stub that toe (let alone, die); but, he says, if we examine the contents of our *conscious* mind, we may realize we were angry with ourselves about something or possibly held the belief "I am a clumsy person." (I stress "conscious" because Seth states this is what primarily creates our experiences: our conscious thoughts, not our subconscious ones.)

Often, he says, we accept our beliefs as statements of fact, rather than beliefs about reality.

You take your beliefs *about* reality as truth and often do not question them. They seem self-explanatory. They appear in your mind as statements of fact, far too obvious for examination. Therefore they are accepted without question too often. They are not recognized as beliefs *about* reality but are instead considered as characteristics of reality itself. Frequently such ideas appear indisputable, so a part of you that it does not occur to you to speculate about their validity. They become invisible assumptions but they nevertheless color and form your personal experience. (Roberts 1974:20)

"Childbirth is painful" is a good example of a belief that most people unquestioningly accept as a fact. It is so thoroughly ingrained in the minds of most Westerners that, in almost all cases, it is indeed painful. Women expect it to be painful, prepare themselves for the pain, and consequently experience it as painful.

Often physicians unwittingly act as hypnotists in the hospital, reinforcing the belief that labor hurts. In *Childbirth without Fear*, Grantly Dick-Read writes,

Suggestion of pain is conveyed by the atmosphere of the labor room; it emanates from doctors, nurses and relatives. They believe in pain; subconsciously or consciously they suggest, expect and even presume pain. Upon the sensitive mind of a woman in labor such authoritative [suggestions are] a powerful adjuvant to painful sensations. (Dick-Read 1959:56)

Not all women, however, experience labor as painful. Helen Wessel quotes one woman who reported that she experienced no pain in labor, at all, and was actually unaware that she was having contractions.

From time to time, the nurse would put her hand on my abdomen and say, "Are you having contraction?" And in all truth I would answer, "I don't think so, I don't feel anything." "Well, you are," she would answer, "only you must be so relaxed that you don't feel it." (as quoted in Wessel 1963:245)

Nurse Jane Dwinell tells a similar story in her book *Birth Stories: Mystery, Power, and Creation*:

> I had not noticed her having any contractions—no change of expression, movement or sound. I listened to the baby's heartbeat while the doctor sat on the bed and did the vaginal exam. "Well, now, you're eight, Ariel. How soon are you going to have this baby? Five minutes? Ten? Fifteen?" We all laughed, and Ariel continued to smile, reclining in bed with her legs spread. I kept my hand on her belly and, sure enough, it tightened. I timed the tightenings while we talked—they were every two minutes, lasting a minute. This woman *was* having contractions. "Can you feel that?" I asked as her belly rose up, contracting firmly. "Not a thing," she said.
>
> Three contractions later her waters broke, clear fluid pouring out of her vagina and puddling on the bed. "Here comes the baby!" she said. Without so much as a moan or a groan, she spread her legs further apart, and I saw the bulge at her perineum. She smiled and reached down to touch the head as it began to show. The doctor supported her perineum, Ariel gave a big sigh, and the baby slipped out. She reached down for the baby—a boy—as the doctor lifted him into her arms. (Dwinell 1992:88)

"Amazing," Dwinell says, "I'll never understand why she doesn't feel anything" (1992:89). In spite of witnessing this painless easy birth, several pages later Dwinell writes, "Yes, there is discomfort associated with being in labor and giving birth. . . . It will hurt" (1992:92). Perhaps Ariel, however, chose not to share in that belief.

A good example of how belief affects labor can be found in the case of a nurse who appeared on the *Geraldo* show. (July 10, 1992). An attractive, intelligent woman told the story of giving birth alone in her bathroom one day. With her first baby she had had a difficult, painful, ten-hour hospital delivery. With this one, she said, she felt no contractions but only a sense of pressure. She gave two pushes and caught the baby as it slid into her hands.

What makes this story even more unusual is that the woman didn't know she was pregnant at the time. The baby was full term and weighed more than seven pounds. Both she and her husband had noticed that she had gained ten pounds over the winter, but it didn't occur to either one of them that she might be pregnant. Unlike her first pregnancy, she had not experienced morning sickness or discomfort of any kind.

After they got over the initial shock, they came to the conclusion that this was the way God had intended birth to be. She felt that, if she would have had conscious knowledge of the pregnancy, it wouldn't have gone as smoothly as it did and she certainly wouldn't have chosen to do it alone. The bottom line is, she wasn't *expecting* pain and consequently didn't experience any.

Nancy Wainer Cohen and Lois Estner, whose book *Silent Knife* (1983) has been called the bible of Cesarean prevention, write that many women do not have beliefs conducive to normal childbearing. If a woman is confused and insecure, she is more likely to have a Cesarean—regardless of her physical makeup—than a woman who is confident and self-assured but technically not so well built for giving birth.

Lester Hazell, the former president of the International Childbirth Education Association, believes that "what happens at birth tends to be guided by our belief system about birth" (quoted in Jones 1987:32).

Childbirth educator Carl Jones writes in *Mind over Labor*,

> A positive image of birth is the cornerstone of a safe, happy birth experience. If you believe your body is meant to give birth efficiently, naturally, and without complications and that birth is a joyful event, you are more than halfway to a safe, natural birth. Positive beliefs and attitudes contribute to a happy birth experience, enabling the mother to labor more efficiently and to open for her baby with less effort. (Jones 1987:32)

Dr. David Stewart, executive director of NAPSAC International (the InterNational Association for Parents and Professionals for Safe Alternatives in Childbirth), is also convinced our beliefs about birth have a profound effect on our labors:

> Although my wife, Lee, felt some anxiety from time to time in pregnancy, the closer it came to the time for labor, the less fear

she felt. During labor she felt no fear at all. This was to a great extent the result of consciously working to clear her mind of all negativity and doubt as well as sending positive and loving thoughts to her unborn child throughout pregnancy. The result was a fear-free, complication-free birth in five pregnancies out of five. Though we coupled our mental and spiritual efforts with excellent nutrition and physical exercise, the fundamental factor in our bearing healthy babies was not of the body, but of the mind. (quoted in Jones 1987:45–46)

Outside of the arena of childbirth, numerous authors have written about the power of belief. Michael Talbot, in his book *The Holographic Universe* (1991), gives instances of people walking through fire and across hot lava without being burned or experiencing pain of any sort. He writes, "The ability of consciousness to shift from one entire reality to another suggests that the usually inviolate rule that 'fire burns human flesh' may only be one program in the cosmic computer, but a program that has been repeated so often it has become one of nature's habits" (1991:137).

What we have actually done, Talbot says, is hypnotized ourselves into believing that human flesh burns. When we choose to believe it doesn't, that then becomes our experience.

On the other hand, William Corliss gives examples in his book *The Unfathomed Mind: A Handbook of Unusual Mental Phenomena* (1982) of hypnotic subjects who produced blisters on their skin after being told they had been burned. In reality, however, they had not.

Corliss also relays the stories of several women who were able to enlarge their breasts through visualization. In one case, the woman realized that her unusually small breasts were due to her desire to remain a child. When she was able to overcome her fear of womanhood, she was able to enlarge her breasts significantly, simply through suggestion.

Pat Carter tells the story of the well-authenticated experiment conducted by French scientists on a prisoner during the Reign of Terror. After telling the prisoner they were going to bleed him to death, they took his arm and put it through a small opening in a wall. The scientists then proceeded to run the back side of a knife across his wrist—an action that did not even scratch the skin—and pour a trickle of warm water down his arm. In a short time, he was dead. An autopsy showed drained and whitened tissues as if he had died from hemorrhage.

Several years ago there was a story on TV about a man whose foot had been completely crushed in an accident. To the amazement of his doctors, through visualization he was able completely to regenerate the bones in his foot.

Soon after seeing this, I went to a dentist and was told I had eight cavities. I decided to hold off on having them filled and instead began visualizing the holes being filled in. If a man could regenerate bones in his foot, then surely, I thought, I could regenerate holes in my teeth.

I told myself that I loved my teeth and was no longer attacking them. (As a child and adolescent I usually had six to eight cavities every time I went to the dentist. My mother said it was probably because there was no fluoride in the water in Connecticut when she was pregnant with me. Years later it occurred to me that my second set of teeth came in while I was living in Denver where there *was* fluoride in the water. My new teeth continued to rot at the same rate.)

I decided to wait a year before returning to the dentist. During that time I realized that I produced holes in my teeth in the same way that some people produced holes in their stomach. I made a conscious decision to stop being anxious about my life and to trust that it would all work out.

I also realized that my habit of attacking my teeth probably originated in my childhood as a response to my tendency to overeat. I had hated myself for this and, in some perverse way, had undoubtedly decided to destroy my teeth so that I couldn't eat.

A year after my appointment, I finally returned to the dentist. Once again he took X rays so that he could "fill the worst ones first." Holding up the X rays he said, "What did you do? Five of them are gone." He held up the X rays from the year before and put them next to the new ones. "Here's where the holes were," he said, "and here's where they're not." For the first time in my life I actually enjoyed a dentist appointment.

In his book *Psychic Phenomena* (1967), physician Robert Bradley writes about working with a boy who suffered from severe asthma. As the boy was going to sleep, Bradley gave him direct suggestions that his lungs were getting drier and drier and his breathing was getting easier and easier. It worked; and later on, the boy found he could achieve the same results by giving himself the suggestions.

> He even applied this same self-suggestion later to stop his nose from bleeding, much to the amazement of his soccer coach. When he got bumped and his nose bled he would decline the offer of a cotton nasal pack; curl up on the ground, close his eyes, concentrate and very efficiently stop the bleeding by self-suggestion. (Bradley 1967:131)

Unfortunately, seven pages later, Bradley states that all babies should be born in hospitals because there is a chance some of the mothers may bleed to death! Bradley makes the same mistakes that many others do, and says, in effect, "I create my own reality—but only to a degree."

To prove his point as to the dangers of home birth, he tells the story of a doctor who was asked to sign birth certificates for a group of people who chose to give birth at home without medical assistance. Bradley was appalled that the doctor had agreed to do so, and told him that eventually he would be signing some death certificates as well. Sure enough, Bradley writes, several *years* later a woman died in an unassisted birth. He neglects to mention how many mothers and babies died in the hospital due to unnecessary medical intervention during those same few years.

Recently I read about an ailing woman who had written extensively about the power of belief. She was still alive, but her prognosis was poor. After becoming ill she had employed the services of a nutritionist and a doctor as well as attempted to heal herself through suggestion. Many people would look at this as the sensible approach to take. However, neither she nor her "professional attendants" were successful. The fact that she had employed the nutritionist and the doctor showed she really had little faith in her own abilities. Her beliefs contradicted each other: her energies were divided, and her body paid the price. I've since heard she's died.

I sympathize with people who have a hard time in accepting total responsibility for the circumstances of their lives. Most of us have not been brought up to believe in our own abilities, especially when it comes to maintaining our health. Often we feel more comfortable putting ourselves in someone else's hands.

However, the concept that we create our own reality according to our beliefs has actually been around for thousands of years. It can be found in almost all the major religions.

In the New Testament there are numerous passages attesting to the power of faith and belief.

If ye have faith as a grain of mustard seed, ye shall say unto this mountain, remove hence to yonder place; and it shall remove; and nothing shall be impossible unto you. (Matthew 17:20)

If thou canst believe, all things are possible to him that believeth. (Mark (9:23)

Have faith in God. For verily I say unto you, that whosoever shall say unto this mountain, be thou removed and be thou cast into the sea; and shall not doubt in his heart, but shall believe that those things which he saith shall come to pass; he shall have whatsoever he saith. Therefore I say unto you, what things soever ye desire, when ye pray, believe that ye receive them, and ye shall have them. (Mark 11:22–24)

And all things,whatsoever ye shall ask in prayer, believing, ye shall receive. (Matthew 21:22)

The Bible also contains passages that teach believing or focusing on what we *don't* want will bring *that* about, as well.

The thing which I greatly feared is come upon me, and that which I was afraid of is come unto me. (Job 3:25)

Buddhism, too, stresses the power of our thoughts and beliefs. Gautama Buddha said, "Mind is everything. We become what we think."

Philosophers throughout the ages have expressed similar sentiments. Aristotle said, "A vivid imagination compels the whole body to obey it." Marcus Aurelius, a Roman emperor and philosopher, stated, "Our life is what our thoughts make it." William James, a turn-of-the-century professor of philosophy, psychology, and anatomy at Harvard University, wrote, "The greatest discovery of my generation is that human beings can alter their lives by altering their attitudes of mind." His contemporary James Allen wrote,

Of all the beautiful truths pertaining to the soul which have been restored and brought to light in this age, none is more gladdening or fruitful of divine promise and confidence than this—that man is the master of thought, the molder of character, and the maker and shaper of condition, environment, and destiny. As a being of Power, Intelligence, and Love, and the lord of his own thought, man holds the key to every situation, and contains within himself that transforming and regenerative agency by which he may make himself what he wills. (Allen 1993:11)

Many present-day authors agree. Norman Vincent Peale, a minister and author of numerous books, states, "Thinking is the body of the rocket. Believing is the propellant which carries it to the stars. Thinking is the birth of the deed. Believing makes it happen" (1990:4).

Richard Bach (author of the popular book *Jonathan Livingston Seagull*)—himself an avid reader of the Seth material—says, "We magnetize into our lives whatever we hold in our thought" (1977:3).

Even some professionals in the medical field are beginning to understand the power of belief. Bernie S. Siegel, M.D., a practicing surgeon and author, states, "The simple truth is, happy people generally don't get sick. One's attitude toward oneself is the single most important factor in healing or staying well. . . . Scientists often say you must see in order to believe, but I know you must believe in order to see" (1986:76, 223).

Dr. Edward Jones, a psychologist at Princeton University, believes that "our expectations not only affect how we see reality, but also affect the reality itself" (as quoted in Peale 1990:18).

Assuming this philosophy is valid, it is easy to understand how a lifelong belief in the dangers of childbirth will manifest itself in the form of a difficult labor and delivery.

On the other hand, visualizing and believing in a painless and easy birth will bring that about, as well. On *Geraldo* (November 26, 1992), actress Catherine Oxenberg told the story of the birth of her baby. She claimed that while she was pregnant she continually visualized an easy birth. Her actual labor lasted only two hours—which is almost unheard of for first-time mothers. Geraldo Rivera, the show's host, implied that perhaps this was just a coincidence. No, she insisted, her labor had accurately reflected her beliefs.

Jane Dwinell, says she often encourages women to use visualization when giving birth, as does Gayle Peterson. In *Birthing Normally* Peterson writes,

> Fear, and especially unrecognized life stress, can constrict the life breathing passageways, as well as the birth-giving passageways of the body. Visualizing the labor process with positive suggestion for ability to birth can be instrumental in inspiring a change of attitude in particular women. (Peterson 1981:39)

Unfortunately, Peterson does the same thing that Bradley does, and says in effect that we can take this belief thing only so far. Birth, according to Peterson, is inherently painful. Perhaps we can decrease the pain, but we can't eliminate it entirely. There are also times, she believes, when things "just happen." It is here that I part company with the majority of childbirth educators. Our minds are infinitely more powerful than most of us realize. We have only begun to comprehend the power of our self-conscious thoughts.

One physician told me that 95 percent of all labors are normal and require no intervention. However, he said, because we can't predict which women will fall into the 5 percent of births that aren't normal, all babies should be born in hospitals. By that rationale, suppose 5 percent of all men were rapists. Does that mean we should lock up all men because we don't know which ones might be dangerous?

Actually, says physician Lewis Mehl, (in Peterson 1981) by interviewing a woman during her pregnancy it is possible to get some idea of how her labor will proceed. If she lacks confidence and determination then, chances are, her birthing will be problematic.

I have spoken to women who have given birth at home, visualized a painless birth, and still had painful labors. "This *proves*," said one of them, "that childbirth is inherently painful!" In reality this proves that, although the woman imagined a painless birth, she still clung to opposing beliefs.

Mike and Nancy Samuels write in their book *Seeing with the Mind's Eye* that "unrecognized negative visualizations counteract the effects of a positive visualization that people consciously hold in their mind" (1975:148). That is why it is important for a woman to examine her beliefs thoroughly. It is not enough simply to "think positively" if she also believes, to one degree or another, that birth is inherently painful, or perhaps that the power of belief is just another "New Age" concept.

NEGATIVE BELIEFS

To understand fully how belief affects a laboring woman, we must return again to Gerald Heard's explanations of fear, shame, and guilt in his book *The Five Ages of Man* (1963). Although they are integrally related, I have separated them here for the purposes of discussion.

Fear

When our ancestors lived in the wild, fear served a very definite purpose. For instance, if a hunter found himself in a dangerous situation, the emotion of fear would instantly send messages to his body, telling it either to fight the danger or to run away. Blood and oxygen would instantly rush into the muscle structure, which in turn would give him the power to do what was necessary to survive. All nonessential organs would therefore be drained of blood (and oxygen) so that it could be diverted elsewhere.

This is why people "turn white as a sheet" when they are afraid. The body assumes that the face is not in need of blood and oxygen as much as, say, the muscles in the legs, which—when given that extra blood and oxygen—enable the endangered person to run. In addition to the skin, other nonessential organs include the brain, the digestive organs, and—ta-da!—the uterus.

Grantly Dick-Read wrote that the uterus of a frightened woman in labor is literally white. Pain, he said, is not a normal consequence of labor. It only comes about when the uterus is deprived of its fuel: blood and oxygen. Without fuel, it cannot function—or, rather, cannot function well—nor can waste products be carried away properly. Fear also restricts the natural expulsive movements of the uterine muscles. A fearful woman in labor tightens her uterine as well as vaginal muscles, transforming the painless simple act of childbirth into something painful and difficult.

Peterson adds that, when the "flight/fight mechanism" (as it is called) is activated because of fear, the body ceases to produce oxytocin, the hormone necessary for uterine contractions to occur. This is actually a protective mechanism also, she writes, for if a woman in the wild were in a dangerous situation she would certainly want her labor to cease. For the modern Western woman, however, fear has become an undesirable impediment.

Shame

As we have become increasingly self-conscious, we have developed a belief in shame. To one degree or another we feel shameful of our minds, our bodies, and our sexuality.

The emergence of shame in humankind's evolving self-consciousness is depicted in the Bible in the myth of Adam and Eve. Originally they were in a state of bliss, at one with God: "And they were both naked, the man and his wife, and were not ashamed" (Genesis 2:25). When they became self-conscious—symbolized by eating from the Tree of Knowledge—they became shameful and covered themselves with fig leaves. In reality, humankind did not become shameful. It *believed* that it did, however, and so suffered the consequences.

The woman of today may think she is much too intelligent to believe in the myth of Adam and Eve; however, she may unwittingly cling to a belief in sexual shame since it is most certainly perpetuated by our culture. We are taught from the moment we are born that our sexuality is shameful and must be covered up. Sex researcher Virginia Johnson-Masters stated, "The whole cultural message—subliminal if not direct—is that you shouldn't be sexual" (quoted in Korte and Scaer 1990:27).

Some cultures, such as those in the Middle East, are so dominated by shame that the women must cover themselves from head to toe. Our culture has reached a higher degree of self-consciousness, and so is less adamant about covering up. Still the vestiges of shame remain.

If a woman believes her sexuality is shameful, she will find it difficult to spread her legs and give birth to a child who is the result of sex. However, not only is conception sexual; birth is, as well.

Several years ago I wondered what the difference was between an orgasm and a contraction. In both cases the uterus is contracting. When I called a nurse and posed the question to her, she replied, "One hurts and the other feels good"(!). In researching the matter further, I discovered that the two experiences differ only in intensity. In fact, some women experience labor as a series of orgasms, rather than a series of painful contractions.

In Marilyn Moran's book *Happy Birth Days*, Donn Reed gave the following account of the birth of his baby:

> As the baby crowned, I knew from Jean's look and sounds that she was having an explosive orgasm, which rolled on and on. What a long way from the pain and agony of conventional myth! Years later we asked a sympathetic doctor about this. "Yes," he said, "I've seen it a few times. It may even be that many women have orgasms during birth, but interpret them as pain because the sensations are more intense than anything previously experienced and because women are conditioned to expect pain." (quoted in Moran 1986:34–35)

To this, I would add that contractions are experienced as painful because we are taught to believe sexuality is shameful and has no place in the wholesome act of childbirth.

In a letter to *Two Attune*, a woman wrote about making love to her husband while in labor: "My water bag broke right after that and I progressed rapidly. Talk about intense orgasm! This was like millions of little endless ones that climaxed into a feeling of pure and utter love!"(1991, #1:8).

In Helen Wessel's suprisingly sexual book, *Natural Childbirth and the Christian Family* (written in 1963, no less), she writes extensively about the sexual aspect of birth. She quotes one woman as saying,

"It was the most intense orgasm!" (1963:209). Another woman says, "It was ecstatic, wonderful, thrilling. I heard myself moaning—in triumph, not in pain! There was no pain whatsoever, only a primitive and sexual elation. . . . With the most spiraling, fascinating thrill of all, I felt my baby slither out. I wanted to shout with joy" (1963:257).

Carl Jones writes in *Mind over Labor* that "many mothers experience a burning or splitting sensation as the largest diameter of the baby's head passes through the birth outlet. Some actually experience orgasm" (1987:150). The majority of women, however, are unable to experience birth this way.

Dr. N. Kalichman studied the similarities between giving birth and having intercourse. In his article "On Some Psychological Aspects of the Management of Labor," he wrote, "As in intercourse, the ideal may not be attained, and the expression of some of these various natural phenomena may be inhibited" (1951:655). Freeing oneself from shame, therefore, is the next step in the creation of a painless, fulfilling birth.

Guilt

Natural guilt is meant to help us. If we do something that is truly wrong (such as killing someone), natural guilt helps us not to repeat it. Most people in this culture, however, have developed unnatural guilt. We feel guilty about everything from sexual pleasure to financial success. We don't believe we deserve it. This unnatural guilt, Heard writes, is also a result of our emerging self-consciousness.

The concept of unnatural guilt is depicted in the Bible in the Christ myth. Humankind so believed it was bad, it felt it had to sacrifice one of its own to appease God. The modern-day woman may think she has gone beyond believing in original sin, yet she may crucify herself in her own way—for instance, with menstrual cramps during her monthly cycle, and with labor pains while giving birth.

All too often our culture reinforces the belief that suffering is ennobling and somehow a sign of spirituality. Our judicial system often emphasizes punishment and condemnation over rehabilitation and forgiveness, as if the latter just aren't practical.

If a woman in labor believes she is bad for instance, for bringing another life into what she perceives as an overcrowded world, she will punish herself with pain. If she believes all gifts must be paid for by suffering, she will surely suffer. Ruth Hartman agrees. In her article "Changing Beliefs about Birth" she writes,

> People are now starting to look at the importance of belief in the childbirth process, as well as for their health in general. Our belief systems do influence the physical functioning of our bodies, and this particularly applies to the process of labor and delivery. . . . Some women may feel like they need to be punished because of a previous abortion and deserve a hard and complicated birth. (Hartman 1993:1)

We must eliminate all guilt, therefore, if birth is to be a joy and not a punishment.

POSITIVE BELIEFS

Now that we know about what *not* to believe, let us talk about what we *should* believe. What follows is a list of qualities that I feel make for not only a successful birth, but a successful life as well.

Faith

It seems faith has a bad reputation these days. "Men of science" tend to put faith at one end of the spectrum, and reason at the other. How rational is it, however, to believe—as many (if not most) scientists do—that life just appeared out of nowhere for no reason? It seems much more reasonable to believe there is a grand design and purpose to existence.

Faith, however, is more than simply believing in God. It is trusting in the natural workings of the body. In *Childbirth without Fear* Grantly Dick-Read writes, "A woman must remember that faith is not only an ethical and emotional acquisition, but a state of mind which creates within the body physical harmony of the activities of living which maintain the highest standard of health and resistance to disease" (1959:235). Our faith, or lack of it, literally causes us to be healthy or sick.

Several years ago I spoke to a Lamaze teacher about Dick-Read. "I don't like him," she said. "He's too wishy-washy. He believes in faith." True, faith is the cornerstone of Dick-Read's philosophy; but it is a faith based on correct knowledge and, as Carl Jones writes in *Mind over Labor*, "Faith that the power of nature will fulfill its purposes in the life creating miracle, is worth a dozen childbirth classes" (1987:36). Learning how to think correctly is infinitely more important than learning how (supposedly) to breathe correctly.

The Lamaze teacher, too, had faith. Her faith, however, was based on a belief in materialism. We all have faith, says religious writer and minister Don Gossett; what's important is where we choose to put it:

Since God has dealt to every man a measure of faith—and all we need to move a mountain is a mustard seed's worth—we don't need to worry about whether we have faith or not. All we need to do is to decide to apply the faith we already have in the right direction. (Gossett 1976:31–32)

The faith that can move mountains is one that is based on a belief in the self and the creator of the self.

Forgiveness

I don't believe the Bible is "God's Word" in the way that fundamentalists do. It was written by men. However, men can be divinely inspired at times. Therefore, I do believe that it teaches some very valid concepts. Forgiveness is one of them.

And when ye stand praying [notice it says "stand," and not kneel or grovel, forgive, if ye have ought against any: that your Father also which is in heaven may forgive you your trespasses. But if ye do not forgive, neither will your Father which is in heaven forgive your trespasses. (Mark 11:25, 26)

I interpret this passage to mean that, if a person doesn't forgive, his or her life will be its own punishment. As the poet George Herbert wrote, "He who cannot forgive breaks the bridge over which he himself must pass." Bitterness and hatred can literally destroy a person, both mentally and physically.

Physician Bernie Siegel gives numerous instances in his book *Love, Medicine, and Miracles* (1986), of people who have healed themselves of supposedly terminal cancer by letting go of hatred they have been harboring toward themselves and others. Ina May Gaskin writes in *Spiritual Midwifery* (1978) about a woman whose labor had stalled until she realized she was angry with the child's father, who had deserted her. When she was able to let go of her anger, she was able to let go of her baby. This is because hatred consumes our energy, and forgiveness frees it.

Hope

Hope is the expectation that our faith will be rewarded. It is the opposite of cynicism, dread, and despair.

Today, many people speak of false hope. If we are realistic, they say, we will not believe in miracles. Isn't life itself a miracle, however? Perhaps hope has been planted in us as surely as seeds have been planted in the earth. If a seed can grow into a beautiful rose, is it unrealistic to have hope that our dreams can become reality? "You are never given a wish," writes author Richard Bach, "without also being given the power to make it true. You may have to work for it, however" (1977:120).

People fear hope because it makes them feel vulnerable. It is true that, if we don't hope for anything, we can never be let down; but we can't be let down because we are already there. Hope, it is said, is a thing with feathers. It lifts us up as surely as the wings of a bird. When we combine it with faith, we are sure to reach our destination.

Patience

Patience, writes Gerald Heard, is a creative waiting. It is not a lying about, waiting for destiny to do its worst. Instead, it is a trusting that, in time, what we have desired will come to pass.

Humankind has achieved so much because, out of all the animals, we take the longest to mature. The colt walks within minutes of its birth; the human, within many months. This period of extended teachability allows us to grow psychologically. We are vulnerable, in a sense, because we are forced to be dependent on others. It is precisely our vulnerability, however, that opens the door to deep and enduring love.

Heard writes in *Prayers and Meditations*:

Our impatience with Nature, with our fellows and with ourselves, is always spoiling the beauty of design God would otherwise show us every moment. All work has its rhythm: wine, wood, stone, all have their tempo, the time they take to season, to mature. And most of all, our souls. (Heard 1949:71)

Persistence

There is a saying that the Devil's chief weapon is discouragement. "The unpierceable armor against that weapon," writes Heard, "is Persistence" (1949:133).

All too often we start out on our path full of enthusiasm and commitment. When we begin to encounter resistance, however, many of us simply give up, unaware of how close we may have been to reaching our goal.

Persistence is the sister of patience. Patience alone will not carry us through. We must be persistently patient if we are to accomplish our goal.

Humility

What's mistakenly called "humility" these days is often a form of egotism—"an absorbed interest in our self-importance if only because of what we take to be our incomparable nuisance value" (Heard 1949:66–67).

True humility is based on self-respect. It is having enough confidence in ourselves to be able to admit that there are others in this world whose knowledge surpasses our own.

On a spiritual level, humility means opening ourselves up to the knowledge within. To be truly humble we must free ourselves from arrogance and acquiesce to our inner selves.

Love

Love is often confused with idolatry. We place the objects of our affection on a pedestal and claim they are something that we are not. True love, however, necessitates loving ourselves first—not in an egotistical sense, but in a humble self-respecting manner.

"Love thy neighbor as thy self," it says in the Bible (yet), most religions look down on self-love. Perhaps this is because they know the power that self-love brings to an individual. For when we love ourselves, we allow ourselves to receive abundance in every area of our lives. It is only when "our cups runneth over" that we have enough to share with others.

Some "men of the clergy" claim we *must* love our neighbor—as if it is something contrary to our nature. Even if this were so, love is not something that can be coaxed or forced. Rather, it is something that flows through all life. When we cease to restrict its flow, we find ourselves both loved by others and able to love them freely in return. As Washington Irving said, "Love is never lost. If it is not reciprocated, it will flow back and soften and purify the heart."

Courage

"Courage," said Winston Churchill, "is the first of human qualities because it is the quality which guarantees all the others." When we decide to take our lives into our own hands, we must be prepared to encounter resistance. There will always be those who believe we are not qualified to do so.

One's most formidable opponent, however, is generally oneself. If we can stand up to our own fears and apprehensions, we will have little trouble confronting those who oppose us.

Most people would agree that these qualities are admirable and perhaps necessary if we are to create the life we desire. But what do we do when we feel that we simply don't possess them? Even is we do possess them, how can we use them to achieve our goals?

In *The Nature of Personal Reality* Seth says, "To act in an independent manner, you must begin to initiate action that you want to occur physically by creating it in your own being. This is done by combining belief, emotion and imagination, and forming them into a mental picture of the desired physical result" (Roberts 1974:121).

The first step to creating what we desire is to believe that it is possible. The next step is to imagine that it is already a part of our reality. Daily visualizations, combined with belief suggestions or affirmations, are the tools we can use to change our lives.

For instance, when I was pregnant, every day I said to myself, "I believe in my ability to give birth painlessly and easily. I believe I am deserving of a good birth. I believe I am not ashamed. I believe I am not guilty. I believe I am not afraid. I believe I love and forgive myself." I came up with numerous belief suggestions dealing with all different aspects of my personality. Then I vividly imagined myself having the kind of birth I desired.

I refused to take the "realistic" approach and focus on all the things that could go wrong, and instead focused on what could go right. I wasn't ignorant of my body's basic physiology; however, I didn't concern myself with the technical aspects of birth. (Physicians, for instance, have an intellectual understanding of the process of digestion, yet it doesn't prevent them from having one of the highest ulcer rates of any profession.) I never imagined myself timing contractions or checking to see how dilated I was. I simply had faith that my body would give birth in its own time. Consequently, the births went according to my desires.

This philosophy works equally well in other aspects of our lives. We identify what it is we wish to achieve, we believe it is possible for us to achieve it, we imagine it is already a part of our reality, and we patiently wait for it to manifest in our day-to-day life. In *The God of Jane: A Psychic Manifesto*, Seth states,

Faith in a creative, fulfilling, desired end—sustained faith— literally draws from [the universe] all the necessary ingredients, all of the details, and then inserts into [physical life] the impulses, dreams, chance meetings, motivations, or whatever is necessary so that the desired end then falls into place as a completed pattern. (Roberts 1981:13)

Of course, we cannot simply sit back and wait for our ship to come in. As Seth says, the inner self will supply us with the *opportunities*, but we must be intuitive enough to recognize them. This is where our dreams and impulses come into play.

Chapter Six

Dreams, Impulses, and Intuition—Our Psychological Lifeline to the Inner Self

Seth maintains that our inner knowledge usually merges so smoothly with our present concerns that we seldom recognize its source, yet it provides the individual and the species with a reliable, constant stream of information through a psychological lifeline to which we are each connected.

—Jane Roberts,
The Nature of the Psyche

The inner self speaks to us constantly, through dreams, impulses, and intuition, gently guiding us in the direction that is most desirable for our continued growth and fulfillment in this world. It knows our goals and desires and lovingly helps us to bring them about. There is a constant give-and-take between the inner self and the conscious mind.

Throughout the centuries, people have looked to their dreams as a source of guidance and inspiration. John Sanford, an Episcopal priest and Jungian analyst, says in his book *Dreams: God's Forgotten Language* (1989) there are more than seventy passages in the Bible that tell of God (the inner self) speaking to people through their dreams. Ancient Assyrians, Greeks, Hebrews, Egyptians, Indians, Chinese, Japanese, and Muslims have all left records indicating they used dreams as a way to receive knowledge from the deeper layers of the self. There is no reason to believe this is no longer possible. We need not be simply passive listeners, however. The inner self eagerly awaits our questions and concerns.

Gayle M. Delaney writes in *Living Your Dreams* (1988) about a process called "dream incubation." This is where we suggest to ourselves before going to sleep that we will have a dream providing us with a solution to a particular problem. Delaney claims her patients are successful at implementing this process on the average of eight out of ten tries.

I regularly use dreams to help me gain insight into various aspects of my life. Once, when I was trying to decide whether to start a new job or return to one I had held several years before, I suggested to myself that I would receive the answer in a dream. That night I found myself working at my old job. I was bored and unhappy. I then dreamt I had started the new one and knew this was where I belonged.

Dreams can also offer us a wonderful vacation from the stresses and strains of waking life. As a child I used to travel frequently; however, in my twenties I had neither the time nor the money to do so. My nightly adventures at that time, in Europe, Hawaii, and even on the moon—made my somewhat monotonous daytime experiences more bearable. I've also vacationed in other time periods, in my dreams. I've been to California in the 1800s and traveled through Germany in the 1920s.

Sometimes I use dreams to experience things that are relatively impossible to experience in my waking life. Once when I was driving in to the valley and the mist hung beautifully over the mountains, I suggested to myself that I would dream of dancing weightlessly through the clouds. An hour later I found myself looking down on the city as my "body" effortlessly and gracefully moved through the night sky. I awoke feeling as if I had actually done it. According to Seth's teaching, I probably had. Consciousness, he states (Roberts 1979), is independent of the physical body and we all travel out of our bodies every night. When we're not afraid, we can remember our adventures.

Another time, I suggested to myself that I would go over the rainbow. I had been watching *The Wizard of Oz*, and wanted to experience my own version of the land of Oz. When I awoke, I remembered crossing a river and realizing I was in Oz. The flowers were bright and beautiful, and the feeling I had matched the way I used to feel as a child when Dorothy emerged from her house and realized she wasn't in Kansas anymore.

Dreams are more than mere entertainment, however. Many inventors, writers, and artists say they have been inspired by their dreams in many meaningful and practical ways. The famous composer Richard Wagner wrote his music in his dreams. William Coleridge is said to have a written the poem "Kubla Khan" in a dream. While writing it down the next morning, he was interrupted by a visitor, conversed about business for an hour, and was never able to recall the rest of the story. Hence, "Kubla Khan" has remained but a fragment.

Professor A. C. Armstrong, Jr., of Wesleyan University, conducted a study in 1892 that dealt with dreams and their ability to help students process certain information. One student wrote,

In my senior year at college I had an essay to write that troubled me unusually. After trying to decide upon the subject and analysis until quite late, I fell asleep and dreamed not only of the subject and analysis, but of all the details. The next morning I wrote out what I had dreamed, and found it far more satisfactory than anything I had ever done in the same line before. Two years before I had exactly the same experience about an equation in algebra which I worked out correctly in sleep. (as quoted in Corliss 1982:370)

Another student wrote,

Have worked out many algebraic or geometrical problems during sleep. Have, when some years ago in Worcester Academy, scanned some fifty or seventy-five lines of Virgil not yet translated, except ten or fifteen lines; felt tired, went to bed, in sleep accurately translated, all of it, and remembered it on waking. (as quoted in Corliss 1982:370)

Many of the concepts that have appeared in this book have come to me in dreams. For instance, in Chapter 3, I hadn't planned on writing about imprinting and its connection to early hospital experiences. After dreaming about it extensively, however, I decided it was important enough to include.

In childbirth specifically, our dreams can tell us the position of the baby, the sex of the baby, the day it will arrive, the best position for delivery, and any other concerns we may have. Judith Goldsmith writes in *Childbirth Wisdom from the World's Oldest Societies* (1990) that tribal women often depend on their dreams to tell them both the sex and the type of personality their unborn children will have.

Dreams can also reveal to us any limiting beliefs we may have that could possibly prevent us from having the birth we desire. Limiting beliefs are ideas we have about ourselves or life in general that are not based on truth. "Childbirth is inherently dangerous" is an example of a limiting belief. "I'm high risk" is another. (I would have been classified as high risk with at least two of my babies, and yet both of them were born easily.)

When we realize we hold a belief such as this, we need only to remove it from our minds and replace it with a more desirable one. Seth says in *The Nature of Personal Reality*, "Think of a limiting idea as a muddy color and your life as a multidimensional painting that is marred. You change the idea as an artist would his palette" (Roberts 1974:34).

Often it is helpful—when attempting to rid ourselves of a limiting belief—to think in symbolic terms. For instance, if we imagine our mind as a beautiful garden,the limiting belief could be a weed that we simply pull out. The belief we desire could be a flower seed that we plant, water, and allow to grow. We can then use our dreams to check on the progress of our new beliefs. In time, they will manifest in our waking reality.

We must remember, however, that the inner self also uses symbolism to convey information. Not all dreams are literal. If we dream we are giving birth to a poodle, we shouldn't instantly inform the media. Instead, we should ask ourselves what a poodle means to us. Some dreams are like psychic newscasts, giving us valid information about ourselves and others. Others are like movies or plays, creatively presenting us with our beliefs in symbolic form. It is up to us to use our intuition as well as our rational mind to interpret the messages presented.

Eileen Stukane, author of *The Dream Worlds of Pregnancy* (1985), gives numerous examples of dreams that reveal women's beliefs about birth. One woman Stukane interviewed told of having a dream during her pregnancy in which she was lying on a table in her doctor's office and somehow peeking inside herself to see her unborn baby. The woman felt guilty about doing this, as if somehow it wasn't her place to look. The doctor then came in and removed the baby through the woman's belly rather than her vagina.

When the woman went into labor several months later, she ended up having a Cesarean. Some might see her dream as precognitive. However, if the woman could have dealt with the belief the dream revealed—namely, guilt about her right to own her own body—she might have been able to give birth vaginally.

Often, Stukane writes, women do have precognitive dreams while pregnant. One women dreamt she had given birth to a baby with a deformed face. In the dream she was horrified and ran screaming through the hospital. A friend appeared and told her she must not deny the baby. When the woman actually did give birth, her baby had a cleft lip. The woman said she felt the dream had reduced the shock of his appearance. She saw it as both an omen and a form of preparation.

In addition to dreams, the inner self also sends us impulses to move in a certain direction. Once again, the urgings are gentle and suggestive, rather than demanding and overbearing. In *The God of Jane: A Psychic Manifesto*, Seth states,

Despite the beliefs and teachings of religion and psychology, impulses are biological and psychic directional signals meant to nudge the individual toward his or her greatest opportunities for expression and development privately, and also to insure the person's contribution to mass social reality. On a biological basis, impulses are like emotional instincts, individually tuned, so that *ideally* they are stimuli toward action that results as a consequence of complicated "inner" computations. These computations are made by drawing upon the psyche's innate knowledge of probabilities on a private and mass basis.

The authority of the self has been so eroded by religion, science and psychology itself that impulses are equated with anti-social behavior, considered synonymous with it, or with

individual expression at the expense of social order. It should
go without saying that impulses are the basis upon which life
rides, and that they represent the overall motivating life
force. . . . Your impulses will automatically provide you with
the proper balance of solitude and company, private and
public activity, exercise and rest, *for you*. (Roberts 1981:17–18)

The concept of the impulses' being like emotional instincts is
certainly an interesting one. No one questions the fact that animals
have instincts. The bird knows how to build a nest, lay its eggs, and
raise its young. Does it make much sense that humans would not
have some sort of inborn instincts also? Would God or nature
endow all animals with instincts to help them survive and give
birth to their young, but somehow forget about humankind?

It makes much more sense to believe—as Gerald Heard (1963)
and Seth (Roberts 1981) do—that we too have instincts. We also
have, however, the free will to discard those instincts if we so
desire, out of fear and ignorance.

The truth is, as much as some physicians claim we "lay people"
are ignorant of our bodily processes and need their expert advice
and direction, we do in fact know how to live our lives and birth
our babies.

As we begin to learn that we can indeed depend on both our
conscious mind and our inner self, our dependence on external
authority naturally diminishes.

Chapter Seven

Stories of Unassisted Births

Birthing without medical assistance is accomplished not by some willful eccentricity, but with the natural strength and sanctity that issue from unbroken trust in the process of life. Enablement comes from doing, merging inspiration and action into a whole. . . . The roots of fear are manmade, but the roots of intuition go deeper than that; following one's heart unfetters the potential to become an artist in the greatest sense of the word.

—Stephen and Kathy Lanzalotta
in *Two Attune*

In 1977, writer Marilyn Moran started a newsletter titled *The New Nativity* for couples whom she calls "do-it-yourself home birthers." Over the next fourteen years she printed numerous articles related to unassisted home birth, as well as birth stories from more than two hundred couples who successfully gave birth without medical assistance. In 1991, she turned the newsletter over to Kathy and Stephen Lanzalotta, who have subsequently changed its name to *Two Attune*.

In 1981, Moran published an excellent book titled *Birth and the Dialogue of Love*. Its basic premise is that couples are perfectly capable of delivering their own babies. Birth, according to Moran, is a personal sexual experience that should be conducted in the dimly lit seclusion of the couple's own bedroom.

Moran believes that hospitals can be dangerous places not only for mothers and babies; she feels that fathers, and the marital relationship itself, suffer as well. Fathers, she believes, should be an integral part of the birth process, just as they were an integral part of conception. When they are denied the right to participate fully, often their feelings toward the infant are ones of jealousy and resentment, rather than love and adoration. However, Moran claims, these negative emotions are misplaced. In an article in the *Pre- and Peri-natal Psychology Journal* titled "Attachment or Loss within Marriage: The Effect of the Medical Model of Birthing on the Marital Bond of Love," Moran states,

> It's not the baby who robs Dad of his sexual partner, causing him pain and confusion; rather one must conclude it is the obstetrician, the self-appointed surrogate for the father during the conjugal act of birth, who actually does it. (Moran 1992:278)

She quotes the following doctor's testimony to this:

> Looking back I know I was guilty of stealing the show from many fathers. I shall never forget the look of rejection on the face of one particular father who was severely reprimanded by his wife for touching his newborn daughter as mother and daughter were wheeled out of the delivery room. (quoted in Moran 1992:277)

When a father delivers his own baby, Moran says, he is emotionally bonded not only to the child, but to his wife as well. She cautions that the father should not become a pseudo-obstetrician, however. She sees no need for timing contractions and measuring dilation. Faith, love (both physical and emotional), and patience are the ingredients that make for an easy, safe delivery.

The following stories from do-it-yourself couples were originally printed in either *The New Nativity* or *Two Attune*. Several of them also appeared in Moran's *Happy Birth Days* (1986) or *Birth and the Dialogue of Love* (1981). I found all of their accounts to be truly unique, beautiful, and inspiring.

Still, there is room for improvement. Most of the women were not able to eliminate pain entirely. Considering the culture most of us have been raised in, this is totally understandable. Hopefully the next generation, however, will take birth one step further, by eliminating all fear, shame, and guilt. Only then will childbirth be experienced as the painless, emotional, sexual, and spiritual event it was meant to be.

A Bond of Admiration and Love
Carl Norgauer
Burbank, California

I am honored to be asked to tell about my experience with home birth and thankful for those working to teach couples how they can make childbirth one of the most joyful experiences that God has given us to know. Indeed, in childbirth experienced as a loving and supportive encounter we reach such a pinnacle of joy that we feel we have become partners with God in the act of creation.

It was in 1966 that my wife, Anka, was pregnant with my first child, Lilana. As you know, that was a time when home birth in the United States was virtually unknown. A few isolated individuals were aware of the dangers and problems of hospital birth, but almost all of us were indoctrinated with fear about the alternative. Midwives were very few; sympathetic doctors rare.

But I knew I didn't want my child to be born in the hospital. For me, to have her born there represented a betrayal of her birthright, an abandonment of my responsibility as a father and a giving up of my commitment to her health and well-being and to our relationship. I knew that for her to be born at home was as normal as for a bird to be born in a nest. I believed in her safe birth as I believed in her potential for healthy growth to womanhood.

Thus, while Anka was pregnant, I tried to find a midwife or a doctor who would come to our home. We found none. In the meantime, however, we read about the Lamaze method and Grantly Dick-Read's book and saw a movie of an actual birth. Most encouraging, however, was hearing about and meeting another couple who had a home birth. It was very satisfying to hear about their success. And we became more resolved about home birth than ever before.

Anka went into labor before we could locate a birth attendant. But she felt well and in good control and we proceeded together with inspired confidence.

Anka's back pains were intense, so I spent most of her arduous labor massaging her back. I worked so hard and long on this massage that I was dripping wet from sweating.

After four hours of labor, Lilana finally slid out to my waiting hands. She was delivered to her waist, and as she paused, she wrapped her little hand around one of my fingers and held on tight, forming at that moment a bond of mutual admiration and love that will endure 'til I die.

Moments later she was all the way out and announced her arrival with a robust, housewarming cry. What a joy! We had partnered with God a beautiful, healthy child.

After waiting a little time for the blood to empty from the cord, I tied and cut it and put our eager baby to her mother's breast. My joy was complete.

The placenta was delivered into the toilet about an hour later. There was some tearing which healed by itself.

We had no knowledge of facilitating techniques such as perineal massage and lovemaking. But for months afterward we were in a state of exultation and euphoria. This tremendous birthing experience developed a great momentum for bonding, nurturing and loving and was the high point of my life. (*New Nativity* 1986, #37:3)

Damian's Birth—A Story of Love and Magic
Caroline Kuijper
County Roscommon, Ireland

Today is Sunday, the beginning of May. Outside our large kitchen window, in the pram lent to us by a kindly neighbor, is our newly arrived son, Damian, not yet three weeks old. He is sleeping peacefully, enveloped by the scent of sweet-smelling wallflowers while being lullabied by the joyous spring songs of the many birds in the bushes and trees around here in this part of Ireland.

His birthday was truly a most wonderful day, a day filled with peace and magic. In my mind's eye, I can still see ever so clearly little Damian being welcomed by an over-joyed Michael, his father, who received our son into his own hands as he emerged from the birth canal, while his 2 year old sister, Joleen, stood by the side of Michael seemingly transfigured by the majesty of this most miraculous of moments.

No "outsiders" were present at Damian's birth. It was a truly shared, intimate family event. That it should be like this was something that I had for long wanted. Over the previous months as Damian grew within me there had also grown an ever stronger intuition that a home birth of such a kind was the most appropriate situation for the arrival of Damian into the world. I really wanted this particular birth experience to be a natural life-positive event, fully shared with those loved ones, Joleen and Michael, who are so intimately linked with me during this part of my life. Being very much in tune with the rhythms of my body and my feelings of all kinds, and knowing intuitively that all would be well, I had complete trust and faith that the outcome would be a most happy one. I felt it to be a tremendously important step to take the full responsibility for the birth into our own hands, to allow the birth experience to develop naturally in the light of the faith we have in ourselves and in the essential goodness of the world, however much it may appear to be permeated by evil and negativity. Above all, I wanted to show how a woman in this age of anti-life technocratic birthing can still bring new life forth in a homely atmosphere of closeness, joy and magic—a real break with current life-negative practices through which most mothers have to give themselves into the cold, clinical hands that manipulate the "assembly lines" along which women are passed in the course of giving birth in the modern "baby-factory" maternity hospitals.

This was not my first home birth experience. Our daughter Joleen had been born here at home some two years before, back in April 1981. Her birth took place in our bedroom upstairs, with our very capable family doctor and his wife present. The memory of her birth is a very happy one, and very special in its own way, as she was my first-born, and everything about the whole event was completely new and awesome.

But since then I've grown a lot and changed a lot as a person. These changes in my person hood are reflected in a greater looseness in my body make-up, in the way I move and hold myself, and in the way I am now so much more grounded than before. I am also much more mature as a woman, with greater self-confidence and ability to act spontaneously in a life-positive way. So all this allowed me to approach the event of Damian's birth in a calm, confident and highly responsible manner, knowing well that my body was now capable of giving birth in a natural way far more readily than before.

In the course of this second pregnancy, I was also much more familiar with the changes taking place within me while I experienced an ever closer awareness of the ever-increasing intimacy with the new human being developing in my womb. A couple of months after conception I had a very clear dream which helped to vastly intensify this feeling of intimacy. For in this dream I was "told" that the coming child would be a boy and that I should call him Damian. This was a wholly new name to me, never having consciously known of this particular name before, nor was any member of either mine or Michael's families called such. So from very early on in the pregnancy my child, though still a foetus,was a person in my eyes, a person whom I referred to by name, as we all did.

While our first child, two year old Joleen, had been born at home there had been several elements involved with her birth that I wanted to avoid if possible on the occasion of Damian's arrival. One of these was the presence of a doctor being so central to the whole event. Another element was that Joleen was born while I was lying in bed. While I could not praise our family doctor more highly, this situation had created a sort of doctor/patient situation with the doctor "leading" and I following his advice. As a result, Michael was unable to play the active and supportive role that we'd both wanted and needed.

I was very lucky indeed to find Dr. Kilgallen when I first came to live here. In his earlier years he had been present at the births of some 2500 children. He liked very much doing home deliveries. And he knew all there was to know about delivering babies. However, just because he was a doctor, my preference was for a midwife to be with me at the time of Damian's birth. I felt that this would make for a closer togetherness between Michael and me while taking the whole birth-event out of the medical sphere altogether.

Try as I might, and I tried very hard, I simply could not find a midwife. And as the months went by I talked much with Michael about the possibility of we being "caught out." Second children can come unexpectedly quickly, and I wanted us to be prepared just in case. But, at the back of my mind I was already planning to call the doctor as late as possible. This was what my deepest felt intuition was telling me and a situation was being created for the birth of Damian and it appeared to me that all I had to do was to just go along with the trend of events and all would turn out well.

Since Damian was due to arrive some time during the Easter holiday weekend when Dr. Kilgallen was off duty, there was also the possibility that I simply would not be able to have a doctor at the birth, in any case. Everything was pointing towards us having to make a joint decision about a "do-it-yourself" birth. I'd fully accepted this possibility all along, since that was what my heart earnestly desired. But Michael was initially unable to share my confidence.

Then one night Michael had a very vivid dream in which he was shown, as if in a documentary film, the horrors of hospital birthing as practiced by modern technocratic doctors. Following this we had a tremendously open and honest talk together, really facing up to all of the real or imagined consequences of a do-it-yourself birth. And over the following days Michael's sub-conscious self disgorged itself of all the fears it had developed about being hurt in the unlikely event of something terrible happening to me. After that, Michael was able to wholeheartedly and enthusiastically accept our shared responsibility in all matters concerning the forthcoming birthing; and we prepared ourselves on all levels for this momentous event in our lives.

A deep peace settled over us, coupled with an exciting eagerness to give of ourselves fully in what was soon to take place.

Preparation for the arrival of Damian included providing ourselves with rubbing alcohol, clean towels, a sharp scissors and disinfectant. At home you don't have to try and create a completely sterile environment. There are no harmful disease-causing bacteria around which one will find in a hospital, for instance. A good standard of cleanliness plus some simple precautions are all that is needed. Our sharp scissors were intended to make it easy to cut the umbilical cord; but, as an American father told us recently, when one of his children was born it all happened so quickly that he ended up biting off the umbilical cord with his teeth when a scissors wasn't available.

Just a few weeks before Damian was born I received a copy of *The Five Standards for Safe Childbearing* by David Stewart. It is filled with a wealth of relevant facts and information about maternity standards together with vital insights into all the elements that contribute positively to or endanger safe child birthing. It really strengthened my belief and confidence about the normality and sheer beauty of having a baby.

One chapter, in particular, fascinated me. Written by Lewis E. Mehl, M.D., it dealt with the importance of belief, how what one believes, and how one's unconscious feelings and motives greatly influence the actual experience of childbirth. After reading this I set about honestly confronting myself on the very deepest levels of my being; and through powerful symbolic dreams, which left me filled with great peace, together with much visualizing a positive outcome to the rapidly approaching birth, I knew that I had no hidden fears or anxieties left.

Another book that influenced me profoundly was *Birth and the Dialogue of Love*, by Marilyn Moran, which I received in the same general period as Damian was conceived. In this thoroughly excellent life-positive book, as well as in her newsletter, *The New Nativity*, Marilyn emphasizes strongly the *sexual-spiritual* aspect of birth, how the birth of a child should be experienced primarily as an *act of love* between a man and his woman. This book also had a big influence on Michael, as did Marion Sousa's *Childbirth at Home* which arrived at the very same time as he was ridding himself of his subconscious fears regarding the coming birth.

A syringe for removing mucus from Damian's throat was provided by our local district nurse. It was not needed, however, so we returned it later with our grateful thanks. After Damian's birth the same nurse said that she'd been praying for a happy outcome to the event. She'd also been asking some older people on her rounds to pray for me as well—for "the young woman who wants to have her baby at home." One old man at hearing this snorted,

"Uh, and what's so special about that? When I was young I remember a neighbor-woman who was going to have a baby. One day she went to the well to get water . . . and came home a while later with the child in the bucket." This amusing story gave me great encouragement, I must say.

Then one night about a week after Easter I had a very odd sort of dream. It was unusual in that it was not "my" dream; and it seemed obvious to me that I had picked it up psychically from Damian in my womb. The dream made it very clear that our son was preparing himself for his first big journey in this life. This helped to greatly intensify the web of magic in which our house was now so clearly enveloped. I knew now that the appropriate situation for the entry of Damian into the world had at last been created. My son, my beautiful son, would soon be in my loving arms. . . .

His actual journey to the outer world began at a quarter to three on the morning of April 14th, when I awoke suddenly knowing immediately that labor had started. Strong contractions were coming in quick succession long and short ones. But they were very irregular, just as they had been with Joleen. I woke up Michael at once. He jumped out of bed straight away, got the fire going in the kitchen and made tea for me and a big bowl of porridge for himself.

Contractions kept coming and going strongly throughout the rest of the early morning hours, with little peace in between. And it took quite an effort on my part to remain really relaxed. But being on our own—in our own familiar surroundings, it was very easy for me to give myself completely to the situation as it developed from minute to minute.

I must say that Michael was a marvelous tower of strength and support, being there close beside me all the time. He provided the all-important stabilizing power, while I was totally absorbed in the mighty birthing process which was so overwhelming. I felt every sensation intensely, pain and the peace in between the pains, the excitement and the tiredness. I was traveling through many emotional highs and lows.

Joleen came downstairs about 7 o'clock. We told her with great delight that Damian was on the way.

From about 9 o'clock onwards or so I began to feel "open" and according to Michael who checked inside, I was open. However, the strength of the contractions seemed to be about the same as earlier and I felt no urge to push whatsoever. At one time I did try to push, but that really felt wrong. So I just stayed as relaxed as possible, letting Nature take her course. This lasted for more than an hour and then I felt strongly, "Now you've been in there long enough. I'm going to help you out. I'm fed up waiting!"

So I stared pushing while Michael supported me as I squatted. Immediately, after one vigorous push I felt Damian coming down. A tremendous excitement filled the kitchen and Michael and I seemed to merge as our eyes met. It was as if we had become one again as we did in a genital embrace. Yes, we were one. It was not just I who was having the baby. Michael was as well. I felt he and I were part of a greater whole, a whole that included also our son Damian and our daughter Joleen. The moment had become ecstatic. Sensations of every kind and color coursed through me. I was one, one with everything. . . .

Then I was conscious of Joleen, standing right by her father, as I continued pushing. And with that I shouted in sheer delight as I felt Damian coming, when I stopped pushing.

Michael was busy massaging my perineum. Everything was going beautifully. Gently Damian's head emerged and for some minutes, which seemed timeless, mucus dripped out of his mouth, as is the way of Nature. It was perfect, just like a dream. . . . Then very slowly he began to rotate and as his face came upwards I felt a tremendous urge—and out he shot, into the safety of Michael's confident hands. There he was!

Damian was born. It was beyond description what I was experiencing—looking at him, touching him, holding him close, and letting him nuzzle at my breast.

Some twenty minutes later we heard someone at the front door. Michael opened it and said, "Welcome, Doctor! I've been expecting you. Our son Damian has just been born!"

Dr. Kilgallen was not a bit surprised when he was told about Michael's psychic message to him early in labor (unbeknown to me). He said that on 14 previous occasions he had gone to a house without being called, knowing that a child was being born there. But while our family doctor was not surprised, I must admit that I was. For a start, I hadn't seen him for three weeks as I'd been expecting to go into labor any time after my previous visit. And when I asked him what made him call at that particular moment, he said that he felt a strong prompting to pay a visit that morning.

The doctor left a little later, knowing all was well. And we—the four of us—were on our own again, getting a chance to adjust to the new situation. And as I sat down to eat a big plate of muesli with whipped cream which Michael had prepared for me, I reveled in the joy of all that had taken place—in the great miracle of Damian's birth in which we had so deeply shared. Yes, it was truly a magical birth. And Damian is a magical child. (*New Nativity* 1983, #26:3)

Three Do-it-yourself Home births
Frances Frech
Kansas City, Missouri

I had my first at-home birth long before it became popular. My son, Brian, turned 26 years old in February. He's a wide-shouldered, long-haired young man more than six feet tall. The second home birth produced Russ, now 22 years old, a tall, slender, red-headed, blue-eyed young man. And the third time around we had Troy Andrew who was 16 years old in August. He's now a fair-haired, brown-eyed, very bright 10th-grader.

I chose to try the home birth route because my hospital delivery experiences had been so unhappy. No one was teaching home birth techniques in those days, so I was pretty much on my own. I did talk to my sister. She's a nurse and delivered many a baby in her long career when doctors arrived too late. She didn't attempt to dissuade me. In fact, she said she saw no reason why I couldn't do it. She did suggest that if I changed my mind at the last minute, I should call the police or the fire department, since the doctor probably would not come!

It was a bitterly cold night, with an ice storm brewing, when I felt the first strong labor pains. I didn't have a lot of things ready, just a pair of sterilized scissors, some string for tying the cord, and a lot of towels.

I can't say for sure how long it took for the actual birth. I remember having several cramp-like pains, followed by a bearing-down sensation. As the baby's head emerged, there was no pain at all, and I now know that the "moment-of-birth" pain that doctors seem to believe is so excruciating is a myth. I called for my husband as the baby was being born and Bob came running into the bedroom.

Brian had the cord around his neck, but very loosely. He was a healthy pink color, his eyes were wide open, and he was obviously breathing, though he didn't utter the expected first loud, screaming wail. In fact, I worried because he didn't cry. He was just lying there looking around as though he were thinking, "Hey, what kind of place is this?"

The birth process had begun around six o'clock in the evening and was all over by 10:30. I remember being intensely hungry, and Bob fixed a bowl of cooked cereal and two slices of toast. I felt wonderful, on top of the world, not exhausted or vaguely discontented or disappointed.

Russ' arrival was about two weeks ahead of schedule. Bob was on a business trip, so he wasn't home when I realized labor was beginning. The contractions were not strong, but I was losing water for several hours. Late that night the strong contractions came. These lasted only briefly before the birth occurred. Russ was pale and obviously not breathing. The cord was over his shoulder and I suspect that during the contractions it had become pinched. I picked him up and slapped him sharply. The resulting cry was the most beautiful sound I ever heard in my life. My baby was alive and screaming.

Troy's birth was as uneventful as a birth can be. I woke up in the middle of the night, knowing that the waters had ruptured. I started to get out of bed just as a strong contraction began. So I lay down again and waited for it to end. Then I reached over and shook my husband, telling him it was starting. I had three more contractions (a total of four) and Troy's head emerged. Seconds later he was out, not crying but breathing and looking around as his brother had. I couldn't wait to hold him, to keep him close to me.

Home birth—its's beautiful!

Incidentally, prior to my home births I had five hospital births and the first one was a cesarean. James was born August 18, 1946.

The section was performed, after 54 hours of labor, due to a brow presentation. As soon as I got to the hospital I was given drugs right away and labored in the bed for 48 hours before the brow presentation was diagnosed. It's too bad I wasn't allowed to labor in a different position, such as hands and knees. But to labor in such a manner was unheard of in those days.

For my next baby's birth I had a different doctor, one who thought it was not necessary to have a repeat section if the circumstances were different from the earlier labor. I gave birth to that baby vaginally only one hour and 20 minutes after my first contraction.

The doctor who delivered my fourth child was a different man, who was angry that I had been permitted to give birth vaginally after a section. He tried to talk me into another section but I said, "Nothing doing!" And I have never regretted it. (Moran 1986:113)

[Frances Frech is the author of *The Great American Stork-market Crash* and *Population Primer*, two books about the myths and facts concerning population. She has appeared on numerous talk shows including the *Today Show*.]

Camille's Birth
Jackie Klassen
Winnipeg, Manitoba, Canada

It was a wonderful pregnancy. I was healthy, well fed, and feeling beautiful with my baby safely tucked in my ever expanding belly. My third baby, my home birth baby. My two boys, ages 8 and 4, were both born in the hospital. The eldest, David, had a birth that was greatly interfered with (epidural block and forceps). Unfortunately, I was young and uninformed at the time. Matthew's birth was much better. I had lists of things to be avoided in the hospital but one hour after he was born, away he went to the nursery. My husband went with him. I was relieved one of us could be with him, but I was left alone to rest [?].

Well, back to Camille. I had the best prenatal care anyone could hope for from my midwife, a very sensitive, experienced, gifted woman.

It was Sunday, August 21, 1988, one week to my due date. I woke up at 6:00 A.M. with leaky waters. I made puddles all the way to the bathroom and sat down. "Plunk," was that my mucous plug? I was getting excited inside, as my contractions slowly started. I had mild ones all day. The waters stopped leaking

We celebrated Matthew's 4th birthday with a party in the park. It was great. When we got home the boys and I had a bedtime snack, corn on the cob and apple slices. I tucked the boys in bed saying, "Maybe we will have our baby tomorrow."

I phoned a friend, Dorothy, just before midnight to come help with my boys if needed, make tea and look after things. She said she would come soon. Then I took a bath. It felt wonderful. I would roll onto my side with each contraction. They were really gaining strength. I found I was slowly breathing through them. It was time to get out of the tub. I phoned my good friend, Roxie, who lives close by, and told her things were really happening. Then a really intense contraction took me. The top of my tummy shook and "Bang," the water was all over the floor. Roxie said, "I think it's time you call Darleen." I thought so too, since she lives out of town. As I was on the phone telling Darleen she should come over, a contraction took my attention. When I got back to the phone it was dead. Darleen was on the way. No more time for phone calls.

Standing in a puddle, swaying back and forth in my living room, I realized there wasn't any more time for people to arrive. I had to change my plan suddenly. Camille wanted to be born. My body wanted to give birth now!

I waddled to my bed, sat in the middle, arms behind me for support and moaned with the down and out feelings. In between contractions I called for my eldest son, David, to wake up. He didn't want to miss his sister's birth.

Sleepy-eyed he asked, "Is the labor starting now, Mommy?"

"Oh yes, the baby's coming now!" I replied. The contractions must have been about 30 seconds apart. David phoned my friend, Roxie, and told her. "My mom is pushing the baby out!" She said she would be right over. David came and sat on the bed.

"Do you see the baby's head, David?"

Calmly, fascinated, and a bit sleepy-eyed he watched his baby sister enter the outside world. She cried a bit to let us know she was okay. "Oh, our baby, David!"

We just soaked up the moments. It was approximately 1:45 A.M. Time came to a standstill. What a wonderful warm, calm, elated state. David brought some clean towels to cover Camille with. People slowly started to arrive. First Roxie, minutes after the birth. David let her in.

A few minutes later the placenta came out. Roxie wrapped it in a towel so that I could move off the messy sheets with Camille. My son, Matthew, woke up and was happy to join in. What a great scene, everyone sharing in the love on my bed.

Dorothy arrived, and sat down and rubbed my feet. At last Darleen arrived, happy to see that all had gone well. She clamped and cut the cord. Matthew was happy to see it really didn't hurt me or our new baby. Darleen checked Camille over. She was fine and healthy, weighing 7½ pounds. She came several times to check on us in the following days.

It was the most wonderful birthing. Everyone helped out so much in the next few days—my mother, Dorothy, Roxie. There was only one person missing, my husband Kelly. We were separated when I was two months pregnant. I wish I could have shared this wonderful event with him.

Camille is 5½ months old now. She is so sweet, happily nursing. I thank God for all my children every day. (*New Nativity* 1989, #50:11)

A Family Affair
Valerie Wiesner
Lake Elmo, Minnesota

The birth of our fifth baby was our first intentional do-it-yourself home birth. We were living in the mountains of Arizona with only one practicing midwife who lived approximately one hour away. That wouldn't allow enough time for her to have arrived at two previous births of ours. So we started planning from the beginning to deliver with only our immediate family present. We felt totally calm throughout the pregnancy, confident we were making the right choice. Birth is such a natural process, and we had experienced four other natural births. We felt so comfortable and confident that we made the decision that if this baby came early, we would *not* go to the hospital, but deliver it ourselves.

The evening the labor started, I wasn't sure if it was true labor or not—it was all so smooth, gradual, and relaxed. Our other children had left with friends for the evening and Joseph and I went out for pizza. Well, the pizza took unusually long and I was getting anxious to get back home and nest. The pizza finally came on its "trusty" (but actually faulty) pizza stand. When Joseph began serving it up, the entire pizza flipped upside down into the bench opposite us. One big hot heap. It seemed unbelievable this could be happening now. No time to wait for a new one. We made the best of our heap and left for home.

The kids arrived about the same time. We told them we thought labor might be happening, but we weren't sure. They headed for bed and I took a bath. It felt like something was happening, but it was light, not intense. I took an enema, thinking that might help things along. About 10:30 P.M. I thought we may as well try to sleep in case things didn't progress for a while. A few minutes after we laid down, I knew we wouldn't be getting any sleep.

We got up and prepared our parlor. This was our favorite room in the house and it had a bathroom connected (and I seem to spend much of my labors there!). Things progressed quickly now. I spent a lot of time on the toilet, as this was the most comfortable place for me. I'd get up and drink lots: water, juice and herbal tea. I also took some homeopathics: Arnica 200 C, and others, which seemed to help. I'd hug Joseph and squat through a contraction, then go back to the toilet; prowling back and forth like a cat, uncomfortable in one spot very long. Joseph kept saying, "I'd better wake the kids," and I kept saying, "Wait, wait, it's not that close yet." But Joseph knows me better in that situation than I do. I honestly felt birth couldn't be that close. Even though it was intense, it was calm and comfortable and peaceful.

Within a couple of minutes of him being pretty insistent on waking the kids and my wanting to wait, I said, "Well, maybe you better wake the kids." The three oldest girls were all up in a couple of minutes, excited and awed. We had covered the couch, and floor in front of it, with an old shower curtain (with papers on the floor) and sheet on the couch. I leaned/sat on the couch edge in a sitting/squatting position and held onto the two older girls' hands. Within a couple of contractions our baby was crowning and then slid right on out. Our youngest daughter sat on a chair opposite the couch wide eyed and in awe. They weren't afraid at all. In fact, the youngest girl, Amber, wants 100 babies!

The birth was extremely clean, hardly any blood, very pure and holy. Our baby was breathing and healthy. It was all so calm and *the* most natural thing you can imagine. We were all so excited. Joseph just had to tease me, and still does, that I wanted to wait to wake the kids and *he knew* it was close! Forrest James weighed 8½ pounds and was 24 inches long.

This is by far the best birth I could have ever imagined and really brought our family closer together. We didn't wake our two year old boy, but he was totally delighted the next morning when he came bounding onto our bed. I told him we had our baby and he had a little brother. He has never been jealous, but very protective and "big brotherly" to him.

I cannot recommend highly enough to have your own baby in your own home with your own family. You couldn't regret it. It's an experience that no couple/family should be deprived of.

We are expecting our 6th baby on October 1st (Forrest is 15 months old) and never hesitated at the thought of another do-it-yourself home birth. We now live in the twin cities in Minnesota where midwives are plentiful and medical coverage easy to obtain. I pass it all up for the best: our family centered birth. *No one* can give me the support that my husband and children can at this most intense time. We all work together and they all love me and help me so much—it is great and fun. I trust my body and my family and, above all, God to see me through this time and we are greatly looking forward to this labor and birth.

Please—try it for yourself. (*Two Attune* 1991, #1:10)

The Best Way to Have a Baby
Aragyn Lutz
Topeka, Kansas

After my wife had two very easy but very frustrating hospital births, I finally consented to having our third baby at home. Our original plans were to find a midwife, but being unsuccessful, we decided to "go it alone."

We had heard of the Birth at Home League and after taking the classes I had a whole new insight to having a baby at home. The training proved to be valuable beyond price, but the mental attitude of all concerned at the classes was the shot in the arm I needed. Finding all the positive energy instead of the negative vibrations we had been encountering was a blessing.

Where can I start telling of the beautiful birth *we* had? Or, shall I say, "love encounter."

When my wife picked me up from work, she told me that "tonight's the night." I believed her because it was her body, and she knew with the others. We had supper, and Moonshadow baked a cake for my birthday which was two days away.

She had been having minor rushes through the evening; nothing extreme, just an awareness of a baby wanting to get out. We let our neighbor take our other two children, and were alone.

Moonshadow felt comfortable walking, so several times we went outside. Inside, I was buzzing around with last minute preparations. Our bed had been made a week before, so all I was really doing was killing time.

At about 9:00 the rushes were getting stronger, so Moonshadow told me to kiss her, and let me tell you—I became really aware! We kissed with each one after that, and I could actually feel the energy that Moonshadow was feeling!

We practiced breast stimulation, and in between rushes sometimes we danced. Moonshadow didn't stay in one position, but moved and changed positions whenever she wanted. We kissed and hugged like we haven't done since we were dating, and I kept assuring her of how well she was doing.

At about 12:10 she was experiencing some pretty heavy rushes, and so decided to get on her hands and knees. I was getting pretty excited by now, and when her water broke in a couple of minutes, I was really ready to explode! Moonshadow decided she would be more comfortable sitting upright against some pillows. Right after she turned over, I got down to see what was happening. I was surprised and thrilled to see the baby's head crowning. I told Moonshadow that I saw the head and she said, "This baby is ready to come out. It wants out," and the next moment the baby's head was out. Not more than one minute later, Moonshadow helped with a little push and the rest of the baby came out into my hands.

I will never be able to describe the feeling that I experienced as I moved the baby onto my wife's stomach. We were both laughing and crying at the same time. I was so excited that I had wrapped the baby up and had not even noted what sex it was. I peaked under the blanket and laughed and cried. "We have another girl." Our second. Nothing I had ever experienced before, or shall after, will match that feeling that night.

Now, one month later, I still look at my baby girl and know that I am the first person to ever touch her. My wife gave me back the gift of love I had given her nine months before. Our love has grown even stronger than before, if that is even possible. To me now, there is no other way to have a baby. I only pray that more people will come to know the joy that I have known by having a home birth.

Moonshadow's account:

Wednesday, August 23rd, at 4:00 P.M. I had a bloody show. I knew we'd have a baby that night. I began having irregular mild rushes at about 5:00. After supper I took a warm bath and lay down for a nap from about 7:00 to 8:00. Then I got up and made a birthday cake for Aragyn. (His birthday was August 25, and I wanted to make sure he had a cake). Still the rushes were mild and irregular.

At 9:00 labor began in earnest. I remember sitting in our rocking chair riding with an intense rush. With the next rush Aragyn came to me and we kissed. It was so tremendous! Half of the intensity left me and I felt suspended! We were one!

During rushes, while kissing, I kept thinking I was a part of nature, a piece of a natural force such as a storm, wave or flower and needed only to ride with this energetic force. I wanted to calmly let nature work me to bring this child to us and physical contact with Aragyn made this calmness possible.

We danced some, while I wasn't on the toilet. I loved sitting on the toilet!

We were always kissing, hugging, and touching. When I felt the baby pressing down we lounged on the bed. I felt the pressure one more time, then my water broke. Aragyn then took his place to catch his gift and with the next rush we were looking at a little gray head! I was so amazed, and knew Aragyn was too, by the brightness in his big blue eyes. With the next rush a baby squirted out of me into Aragyn's hands.

He immediately put this slippery, slimy, little creature on my belly. As I hugged this scrunched-up child we laughed and cried, for there were two small cries and we knew we had a healthy baby. We'd done it! Those moments were so electrifying I can feel the thrill whenever I remember.

About 45 minutes later Aragyn clamped and cut the cord. He took his new daughter and held her close, a joy he'd been denied before.

We were still waiting for the placenta. I had the urge to stand, so I did. A few moments later I delivered the placenta. It was one hour and ten minutes after birth.

It was very exciting the next morning when our 2½ and 4 year olds came home to meet their baby sister. They held her and kissed her. We've never had any jealousy problem.

I wish every couple could experience the joy and simplicity of a natural home birth. It's so nice for the baby and it gave our relationship a new depth. (Moran 1981:192)

Out of Love
Grace Grazyna Karubin
Los Angeles, California

My 7 births, my 7 rebirths, my 7 real Christmases, real loves, real fulfillments . . . I'd like to write about them a little bit, even though I know that words are not enough to describe what is in my heart when remembering these most important events in my life.

Choosing to give birth only by ourselves, heart-to-heart, was sort of natural for our romantic, Polish natures, although at first we were not quite aware of this "soul connection," for it was something normal in our country of great romantics like F. Chopin. Right from the beginning my husband, Jarek, and I perceived our marriage not as a social institution, but as a union of our beings with which our personal differences had little to do. After giving two so-called "natural births" in the hospital to Mark and Zofia, we decided we needed to do it our way. Those two were painful learning experiences. The next five were born in a delightful, intimate way: in our home and only by ourselves.

Agnieszka, our third child, was joyously born in the kitchen (she is a great cook now!). The next two births were boys, Michal and Milosz, and they had seen the world in the bedroom of our small cottage in the mountains of southern Poland, far away from any hospitals or even a telephone! Jarek was actively involved in the Solidarity Movement in Poland and because of his illegal activities, he was arrested and disappeared for 3 weeks shortly before Milosz's birth. I was in tears preparing to give birth by myself when Jarek managed to come back. Milosz's birth became our great, unforgettable reunion. We depended totally on our spiritual inner strength, wisdom and resources and it was fantastic—so beautiful and romantic.

Our 6th baby was a girl, Milka, who was born on the spread towels of our bedroom's parquet floor in an historic building in the center of Warsaw, our beloved home city (a few steps from "The Clinique of Obstetrix" which we never visited or had any wish to!).

Three months later we emigrated to America, leaving everything we had behind, but talking only our most precious "possessions" with us: our 6 children. And here in Los Angeles, our 7th child was born three years after our arrival.

This last birth was truly my "7th miracle," the perfect answer to my prayers, visualizations, affirmations and meditation. It was very peaceful and yet ecstatic, spiritual and sexual. I gave birth underwater after less than an hour of labor. There was no pushing and almost no blood was lost. The placenta slipped out by itself 1½ hours after the birth.

Every time our births happened differently, but with one thing prevailing in all of these (last) births: the need for uninterrupted and uncontrolled intimacy, freedom and closeness in which our love could work miracles. This love—spiritual connection between our beings—has been the most important factor in creating our family in spite of outside problems put between us; teaching us to creatively lead our lives in Everpresent Here and Now with respect to all of life.

What always amazes me is that while there is so much talk all around about love and sex and building healthy relationships, there is so little said about birth. It's as if birth wasn't a natural part of this beautiful process of falling in love and having sex, but rather as if it were some scary, dangerous disease that one can get by talking about it! To me, my pregnancies, births and breast feedings have always been the most important part of my being in love and expressing myself as Woman, as well as being loved by Man in my life.

I believe and experienced that pregnancy, birth and postpartum don't belong by their nature to the medical field. The more I isolated myself from medical thinking and medical people, the better off I was during my pregnancies, births and postpartums. I was able to find my own *inborn* power which was always in me and I refused to give it up by expecting some specialists to take the responsibility for me or my family. God gave my children to me directly, and I am responsible for their development. I find all intrusions in my work humiliating. My intuition is the way by which I can receive guidance from the only real doctor, healer, teacher, friend, lover—also mother, father and child—who is God—the Highest Love expressing itself on all levels.

This very intuition has told me that children should be given birth in the way they were conceived—with love and passion—and I believe all of us, God's magical children, will learn to live this way, too.

Our births have become an enchanting celebration of our relationship with ourselves and with God, the celebration and lesson of Life—of tasting God and it tasted delicious. . . . I was always convinced that when we had given Nature the chance there was no way "something might go wrong"; for I knew it in my heart that God never did and never does plan for failure. I believe strongly that as long as we are able to attune to God's plans, to all natural energies ruling the process, everything goes simply and smoothly in the most safe, harmonious and effective way known to humanity for thousands of years. . . . And we didn't invent it, it was always there—like electricity—but we were not aware of its qualities and didn't know how to use it intelligently and safely.

In order to use this knowledge or let it work, some special conditions are needed: intimacy, safety, closeness, feelings of being loved and admired, commitment, concentration and undivided attention, undisturbed peace and deep relaxation of mind and body. I personally could find those conditions only at home and with my husband. I've experienced 5 times that only with him— without any witnesses—and I was able to surrender and attune intuitively to my female energy—the same one that was uniting me with my husband during the conception of our children. Both processes had the same nature: opening, releasing, giving and forgiving . . . all we had to do was just simply relax and play, allowing Divine Action to take place in its own Order which is beyond our human comprehension. All attempts to control only complicate and disturb. So it wasn't by accident that 5 times the tears of ecstasy were rolling down my face when in the quietness of Spirit my baby had come out of me—out of us—out of love. (*Two Attune* 1992, #5:10)

Chapter Eight

The Case for Autonomous Birth

Autonomy means independence. The term is generally used by social scientists, theologians or psychiatrists to refer to the individuated, self-actualized or authentic human being, a self-governing and self-defining person, subject primarily to his own laws of being and deeply sensed goals and values. This does not mean that autonomous individuals reject social customs out of hand, but rather that their locus of control, their reference point for decision making, rests within. . . . Autonomous persons consciously author their own lives.

—Marsha Sinetar,
Living Happily Ever After

When we truly accept the fact that we create our own reality, all fear of pain or complications in childbirth vanishes. We feel comfortable giving birth by ourselves or in the company of our mates, friends, or family. When no fear is present, some women actually prefer to be completely alone. In a letter to *The New Nativity* one woman wrote, "As long as I was alone and able to yield to the sexual joy of the birthing, I was able to experience wonderful orgasmic feelings and no pain at all" (1980, #4:8).

Solitude, it appears, may actually be beneficial to the laboring woman. When she has no overly concerned observers to "comfort" her, she can be free to look within herself for support and direction.

Physician and author Michel Odent agrees. He believes that "the length of labor is proportional to the number of people around" (1992:23). The more people observing, Odent says, the longer the labor will be. In *The Nature of Birth and Breastfeeding*, he states that almost all animals seek seclusion when in labor. This allows the mother, as he puts it, "to go off to another planet" (1992:23)—or in other words, go into an altered state of consciousness that allows for the safe and easy delivery of the baby. When a woman feels she is being observed, generally she is unable to do this.

In a film by Professor Cornelius Naaktgeboren on the psychogenic factors in animal births, Naaktgeboren talks about observing a rabbit in the process of giving birth. When he first noticed her, she had already given birth to one rabbit. Knowing there would soon be more, he stood with camera in hand and eagerly waited. "Although I waited for over two hours nothing happened, whereas normally the expulsion phase for a litter of rabbits does not take more than about ten minutes. I decided to leave the animal for a short time. At my return, twenty minutes later, I discovered thirteen newborn rabbits" (as quoted in Arms 1975:131).

When sheep are observed and unnaturally disturbed during labor, Naaktgeboren says, contractions are severely delayed and often a veterinarian must be called in to assist.

In *Husband-coached Childbirth* (1965), Robert Bradley writes extensively about animal mothers seeking out secluded locations in which to give birth. He tells the story of his own dog who meticulously lined her basket with soft soiled clothes from the family's laundry basket.

> Wise mother that she was, she was upset by the attention her acts were bringing from the overly interested children and after the household was asleep, cunningly transferred her nest padding to a closet left open in the bathroom. She gave birth to her puppies peacefully and quietly during the night without arousing a soul—much to the disappointment of the children. (Bradley 1965:24–25)

Bradley mistakenly believes, however, that the human female must not give birth alone. "Animal fathers' presence in labor is unnecessary, as the animal mother can rely on her instinctive know-how and needs no coaching. However, your wife, lacking this instinct, must be guided, directed, and encouraged" (1965:22).

Being the man of contradictions that he is, though, Bradley later queries, "Could the religious convictions of my mother and Dr. Dick-Read's patient have caused a serenity which thinned the clouds of anxiety and fear, allowing the automatic guidance of instinct to penetrate? As an obstetrician I have seen this many times" (1965:181).

On the other hand (!), he says, only "prenatal education and guidance coupled with the reassuring presence of the man she loves, constantly coaching and encouraging, [will] allow your wife to function as an instinctive animal, enabling her to joyously give birth" (1965:181).

(I do credit Bradley with helping to reform modern methods of childbirth. He made many wise observations, but—as with Grantly Dick-Read—he just didn't take them far enough.)

Pat Carter, author of the book *Come Gently, Sweet Lucina* (1957), compares giving birth in the presence of others to dancing in front of a crowd of people. When we are alone, she says, often we dance beautifully; but when people are watching, suddenly our talent seems to vanish. Another analogy she uses is being told by the boss to perform a task at work. Perhaps we've done it well, a hundred times before; but when the boss is looking over our shoulder, watching our every move, suddenly we flounder. (Gayle Peterson calls this "performance anxiety.")

Carter wrote her book in 1957, after giving birth to seven children without the aid of a doctor, midwife, or mate. She had been unhappy with the treatment she had received in the hospital with her first two babies, and vowed never to return.

An editor wrote on the front flap of her book that the book could have been called, "How to Be Pregnant and Not Look It." A more appropriate title, in my mind, would have been "How to Give Birth Successfully in Spite of Limiting Beliefs." Carter, who's since died, had some very unusual ideas. She believed a woman should practically starve herself while pregnant, to ensure a small baby. She herself smoked heavily during her pregnancies so as to avoid eating. She also believed a woman should wear a tight girdle or corset throughout her pregnancy to further ensure that her baby would not be too large to fit through the birth canal.

Still, because she believed that birth was a supremely easy and natural occurrence for which her body had been perfectly designed, she was highly successful in delivering her own babies. With two of them, she writes, she had almost no notice of their impending birth. She felt no contractions and barely caught them before they landed on the floor. The problems in birth occur, she says, when we work against nature, rather than with it.

> Actually if there is no opposition from the birth canal and the cervix [due to fear], the uterus doesn't have to work hard. Until the last contraction I cannot tell it is working as a rule unless I place my hand on my abdomen to see if it is hardening. Otherwise, all I feel is a sort of wave coursing over the body, as if things were happening in the bloodstream, and a sort of numby feeling around the abdomen like just before your foot goes to sleep, only when it doesn't. That Uterus doesn't have to kill you with those contractions. They don't have to be hard if nothing is fighting them. But, oh, when it meets opposition, how determined the Uterus can get, and alas, the agony it can bring in accomplishing its ends. (Carter 1957:177–178)

Carter's last birth, which took place when she was in her forties, was attended by Mary Lou Culbertson, a reporter for the *Daytona Beach News Journal*. Culbertson attested to the fact that Carter gave birth as easily as she claimed.

> [Pat Carter's] calm efficiency and quiet happiness during the birth of her third son was something to write about. She permitted me to be present and to take pictures for my newspaper which is how I gained the name, "baby birthing reporter." She agreed to this publicity for the sole purpose of helping other women find the way to easier childbirth. Newspapers everywhere picked up my features by the way of the Associated Press and made world-wide headlines. . . . Mrs. Carter had her baby with ease, dignity and finesse. Except for me, who was busy shooting pictures, there was no one else present. She didn't moan, cry, shriek, gasp, or shudder, as a woman may ordinarily do while having a baby. She showed absolutely no signs of fear or concern. . . . There were no

indications of pain before, after or during the birth by Mrs. Carter. She simply relaxed on her couch and had her baby. (Culbertson, in Carter 1957:x–xii)

As with Odent, Carter believed a woman should obey her instincts and seek seclusion—not out of a mistrust of others, but rather out of a trust of herself.

The greatest of all preparations for pleasant childbirth is entering into and sustaining a state of outgoing love for others. This will come of its own accord, as the prototypal waves of tender emotion toward the unborn child have been presaging ever since the quickening if a woman is given half a chance by friends and acquaintances to let it flower in solitude, or in the bosom of her family alone.

If she goes forth into the world, she is girded for the encounter, the same as an animal that leaves its lair. But any invasion of her privacy is a direct violation of her instinctive need for it that is part of her inheritance from a far distant past when intrusion meant actual danger to her life and her little one's. The impulse for escape surges within her, but she is caught in a trap of civilized mores, and the impulse is frustrated. Her body becomes tense with that frustration, and wreaks its vengeance upon her mind. And she is reduced to tears or anger. (Carter 1957:196)

Giving birth autonomously, as Carter states, does not necessarily preclude the presence of others. What's important is that the laboring woman follow her instincts and give birth in the way that she desires. Odent agrees:

When the mother-to-be is alone with the baby's father and he seems to really share the emotions, leaving our world at the same time as his wife—a scene that would have been considered unbelievable fifty years ago—it is also possible that the birth will not be too long away or too difficult. In this case, once more, nobody behaves like an observer. It is not the woman who is giving birth; it is the couple. (Odent 1992:23–24)

Often, however, Odent writes, a husband may actually cause a woman to have more difficulty in labor, rather than less. He cautions husbands not to prevent their wives from shifting into another level of consciousness. They must not look into the eyes of their wives as if saying, "Stay with me" (1992:24). Rather, they too must fearlessly allow themselves to experience the new and exciting shift in consciousness if they are to make a positive contribution to the birth.

Carl Jones in *Mind over Labor* (1987) gives a good example of a husband who actually added to his wife's problems in labor, rather than alleviating them. After the woman began to moan during a contraction, the husband said, "Don't do that, honey! Breathe with me instead." He then demonstrated a panting breath they had learned in childbirth class, and encouraged his wife to do it with him. Jones writes, "This is poor advice. Telling a laboring woman to stop moaning and instead pant like a dog on a hot summer day can actually impair labor. Forcing herself to focus her attention on controlled breathing takes the laboring woman away from her instinctive self" (1987:27).

When all is said and done, however, birth is still a solitary act—one individual giving birth to another. True, we are all parts of a whole, but we are individuals nevertheless. Only when we lovingly accept and embrace our individuality can we truly perform miraculous acts.

My husband was present when I gave birth to my first and second babies, and I thoroughly enjoyed his company. However, on subsequent births, I chose to be alone because I viewed it as my personal challenge. It gave me the opportunity to depend completely on myself, and I found that indeed I could. What follows is my story.

Chapter Nine

My Story

I was born in the late 1950s and raised in the suburbs. My father was a physician, and my mother a housewife until she began working as a medical research technician when I was fourteen.

Although we celebrated religious holidays, we never participated in organized religion or belonged to a particular house of worship. At times I wished we had because I longed to be fully accepted by the religious community with which we were very much involved. I understood how my parents felt; however, it seemed to me that they threw the baby out with the bath water. Maybe organized religions were not the way to go, but believing God did not exist at all was equally unsatisfying.

According to my parents there was no spiritual reality, no life after death, and certainly no omnipresent, loving, and forgiving God. We were on our own in this world. Sickness and death could occur at any moment; and when life was over, it was over. We had only the cold, hard ground to look forward to.

Images of death haunted me throughout my childhood. Our house backed up to a cemetery and I could see the graves from my bedroom window. *"What's it all for,"* I used to wonder, *"if we're all going to go there in the end?"* I wanted to believe there was something more to life than what I could perceive with my five senses, but somehow I just couldn't imagine what that something was.

My parents saw my sadness but didn't feel capable of dealing with it. They sent me to psychiatrists periodically, but it didn't do much good. The psychiatrists had the same mechanistic beliefs as my parents and so were unable to offer me much hope.

My father was successful in his profession and, to one degree or another, we all lived through him. When my mother finally awoke to the fact that she had little identity of her own, she went back to work. (Prior to having children, she had been a chemist.) Mothering alone hadn't made her happy; and although my sisters and I tried to be understanding, we felt that in some way she was abandoning us.

Looking back I can see that both she and my father loved us, but I think they were unsure in their own minds as to what the secret of happiness was. Maybe it was a new job or a new house or a month-long vacation away from the kids. Somehow we ended up feeling as if we just weren't an important part of their lives.

Most summers we took a family vacation. We went to Europe, the Virgin Islands, Hawaii, and New York, and often we enjoyed ourselves. But always there was an underlying sadness that money, status, clothes, and trips just couldn't shake. I remember being in Europe one summer and thinking, "*I'm halfway around the world and I'm still miserable.*"

School was a major source of frustration for me. My grades were decent but I couldn't stand all the seemingly arbitrary rules—no talking during lunch, girls must wear dresses even on cold winter days, no going to the bathroom unless it was a scheduled class break (I wet my pants once when my bladder insisted on being independent of the rest of the first grade), and a host of other meaningless policies designed to keep us docile and subservient.

At about the age of eleven I began to overeat. Both my mother and my older sister Susan were slightly overweight, and I remember thinking maybe they would like me better if I joined them. Susan and I had never been close before. Now, pigging-out became a social event for us. Maybe she didn't want to play with me, but she certainly would sit down and eat with me.

Soon my weight far surpassed hers. Food became my drug of choice. I ate when I was lonely, frustrated, depressed, or angry. The resulting fat served as a barrier between me and what I perceived as a dangerous, uncaring world.

The fat also hid my emerging feminine figure—which, in some ways, worked to my advantage. Femininity would only lead to contact with men, and that frightened me. Men were impregnators. And pregnancy was a fate worse than death. Motherhood was not to be in my future, I had decided. It seemed not to have brought my mother much happiness—so why would it be any different for me? I loved playing mother to my little sister Janet, but that was the closest I ever planned on getting to the real thing.

Eventually my adolescent hormones took over, however; and at the age of seventeen I lost my virginity to a boy I hardly knew. Our relationship was short lived—due to a pregnancy scare. It turned out that I wasn't pregnant, but just the thought of it had frightened him away.

I longed to tell my mother what was happening, but I didn't dare. Sex was just not something she felt comfortable discussing. As a matter of fact, up until the time I was twelve I honestly thought conception took place while a man and a woman slept peacefully next to each other, fully clothed and unaware of what was happening.

After Pete (the first) and I stopped seeing each other, I proceeded to sleep with numerous other men. None of them cared for me nor brought me much happiness, but it was a new sensation, if nothing else.

The summer before I went to college I gained thirty pounds. A typical day would start out with five bowls of cereal, followed by a morning nap. I cried myself to sleep every day. I hated what was happening to me, but I didn't seem to be able to control it.

Often I would write about my frustrations. However, although it felt good to express myself on paper, I wasn't able to come to many insights. Life just didn't seem to make much sense. Everything appeared to be outside of my control. I was fat and lonely and had little hope of changing either condition. I contemplated suicide many times. But something inside of me always said, "It isn't that bad. Don't give up. Life will get better."

So, in the fall of 1975, I packed up my tent dresses and platform shoes and left for the state university in hopes of starting a new and hopefully better life.

Once I was settled in at school, I was bored with my classes, basically. But I enjoyed living in a dorm and being more independent. My freshman year was fairly uneventful until one February night.

A boy I had been seeing moved into a large house near the campus and I ended up spending many nights there. Our relationship was beginning to deteriorate and, one night after one of our numerous fights, I walked across the hall and began socializing with several of his housemates.

It was an old boarding-type house with about thirty rooms, so I hadn't met everyone yet. As we were talking, a very tall man walked into the room. Everyone seemed happy to see him. He introduced himself to me as David Shanley, and I instantly liked him. Some of the people in the room were joking that David couldn't visit someone in the basement because at six foot eight, he wouldn't fit. David laughed. He was neither ashamed of his height nor vain about it.

He began talking about a subject that had been fascinating him lately: the evolution of self-consciousness. Everyone was interested and we ended up talking for several hours. Eventually people began to leave, but I had no desire to go to sleep. David and I went back to his room and talked all night.

The next morning we went out to breakfast. I remember looking at him as we walked along. His hair was long and black and his features were beautiful. I thought for a moment, *"Would this man ever be interested in fat, dumpy, insecure me?"* Instantly I decided no. Yet, he seemed to enjoy talking to me, so I began visiting him every few days from then on.

David was a senior majoring in history, but his real interests lay outside of school. He had come across Gerald Heard's *The Five Ages of Man* (1963) the year before and was determined to alter his conduct, character, and consciousness, as Heard had advised.

Every morning he awoke at 3 A.M. and began reading an earlier Heard book titled *Prayers and Meditations* (1949). The book dealt with concepts that at that time were totally foreign to me: humility, forgiveness, patience, and persistence, to name a few. Even at the age of eighteen, I literally did not know the meaning of humility. Forgiveness was only for suckers. I didn't want to be patient—I wanted everything right now, and the only thing I had ever been persistent at was eating.

Heard's belief system, however, appealed to me. Life was not an accident, and death was not the end. There was a purpose to all of this. Suddenly a ray of sunshine entered my darkened soul.

David started me on a program of what he called "psycho/physical development." I began reading books, lifting weights, and running. The energy that had once gone into depression and overeating went now into this mind/body training. Soon the fat began to disappear—and with it, my feelings of inadequacy.

The first book I read was Grantly Dick-Read's *Childbirth without Fear* (1959). David had read it after seeing it in Heard's bibliography and was instantly convinced of its validity. Of *course* childbirth wasn't meant to hurt. As I read the book, maternal feelings began to surface in me for the first time.

Meanwhile, conflicts began developing at school and with my parents. In my women's studies class, a teacher gave me a low grade because I disagreed with her statement that "Sylvia Plath committed suicide because she saw too much." "No," I argued, "she didn't see enough. If she would have really opened her eyes, she would have seen that life is not hopeless and meaningless." My teacher, being the "realist" that she was, wasn't impressed with my optimism.

At home, my parents also had no interest in my new found enthusiasm. With tears in my eyes, I said to my mother, "There's some sort of spiritual reality or God. I know. I can feel it." She instantly changed the subject.

In December of 1976, I moved to California. David and I had become lovers the previous July (much to my surprise), but I didn't think I was ready for a serious relationship at that point. I finally had some self-confidence, and I wanted to get out into the world and try my wings.

California was wonderful. I lived in a motel on the beach and worked as a switchboard operator in exchange for my rent. Some afternoons I worked in a little cafe near the motel. I was supporting myself for the first time and I loved it.

When I wasn't working or lying in the sun, I was reading. There was a small bookstore between the cafe and the motel, and most afternoons I would spend at least an hour browsing through it. It was filled with books about Buddhism, spirit guides, and altered states of consciousness. I was fascinated. My landlord showed me a copy of *Seth Speaks* (1972) by Jane Roberts. It looked interesting, but not interesting enough to read. I had plenty of other books to keep me busy.

Most of my nights were spent walking along the beach, thinking. One night as I sat in the sand, listening to the gentle rhythm of the waves, a strange feeling came over me. "*I've made it. I'm grown up. I'm not a little girl anymore,*" I thought to myself. It was as if I had suddenly crossed that line into adulthood and I knew it. I ran in and called my sister Susan, and we both cried.

Four months after I arrived, I suddenly felt homesick, so I packed up my bags and went home. I decided to lived with my parents until I could find a place to live. David was happy to see me and eager to show me a book *his* landlord had given him: *Seth Speaks*. I thumbed through it and decided to read it when I got the chance.

Soon after that, I had a dream that was so intense I awoke with my heart pounding. In the dream, I was living in my great-grandmother's house. For some reason, she didn't live there anymore. Instead, I shared the house with a woman and two men. The woman seemed to be my friend, but I didn't get along well with the men.

Suddenly a giant tidal wave swept over the house. A minute later it was engulfed with flames. Fire raged everywhere. I started yelling and screaming at the girl I lived with, but later apologized saying I was on edge because I had my period.

I knew that no one had been hurt in the fire, but I awoke quite shaken. The dream was so powerful that I wrote it down—something I rarely did.

About two weeks later I ran into an old friend of mine. She said she was living in a small town near where I went to school, and told me to stop by. Several days later I did, and she asked me to move in. The house was lovely. But the two men who lived downstairs were not very friendly. Kim and I got along well, though, and I was eager to be on my own again. So I took her up on her offer.

A few weeks later I was taking a bath and letting the hot water run over my feet. The bath was full, so the water was going into an overflow hole below the faucet. Unbeknown to me, the hole was connected to a pipe that led nowhere. Water poured onto the ceiling of the first floor and shorted out the lights. Sparks were flying downstairs as I peacefully soaked in my bath.

Suddenly one of the men from downstairs came running up screaming at me that I had almost started a fire. I got out of the bath and proceeded to scream at Kim—even though she had said nothing. She stormed out of the house. When she did return, I apologized, saying that I was upset because the man downstairs had yelled at me and that I was already edgy because I was having my period.

Several hours later, as I was looking out the window, I began thinking about how much this house reminded me of my great-grandmother's in Brooklyn. At that point the dream came back to me. I stood there stunned as I recalled the similarities between the dream and the recent events: the tidal wave was the bath water; the raging fire was my raging emotions and the potential fire; my great-grandmother's house was this house that reminded me of her house, and in both the dream and reality, I lived with a woman and two unfriendly men. In both cases, I yelled at my roommate and apologized saying I was edgy because I had my period. The dream had occurred weeks before I even knew of the existence of the house.

For the next few days I thought of nothing else. All it takes is one precognitive dream to shatter one's illusions of what time is and what it isn't. Obviously, I realized, I had a lot to learn.

I began reading *Seth Speaks* and proceeded to have more interesting dreams. In one, I felt myself go out of my body and fly to my parents' house. I was looking at the mail slot by the front door when a letter came through it. It was a letter that my parents had mailed to someone but that, for some reason, had come back. Suddenly I was back in my body and wide awake.

The dream was so real that I called my mother, told her about it, and asked if any letters had been returned to them. She said no.

The next day I went to my parents' house. The mail came and there was a letter that my parents had mailed to my sister in Europe the month before. The letter had been forwarded several times, but my sister had already returned home so the post office had sent it back to my parents.

"Here's the letter I dreamt about!" I yelled

"You dreamt about a letter?" my mother said.

I eventually gave up trying to convince my mother of the significance of dreams. But I learned to take them seriously.

Both David and I were fascinated by what we were learning about our minds. We suddenly felt as if we had been given a new toy. We were filled with childlike wonder and curiosity.

In June of 1977 we began living together. We continued to take classes, but spent all of our free time reading Jane Roberts/Seth books. We were determined to create beautiful lives for ourselves. Both of us were beginning to have strong parental desires, so at the end of the summer I went off birth control. We trusted that, when the time was right, I would conceive.

On November 30, I had a dream in which I was holding the palms of my hands about an inch apart and turning them slowly, as if forming something between them. A brilliant blue spark suddenly appeared before me. I woke up, woke David up, and said, "I feel like I just created something." I went back to sleep and dreamt I was carrying around three babies that were as big as my thumb and I loved them all dearly.

In December I didn't get my period, so in January I went to Planned Parenthood and took a pregnancy test. The technician said I was pregnant and would have conceived around November 30. Several months later as I was looking through my dream journal, I came across the dreams from that night. I realized I had dreamt of my baby's conception. (Since that time I've read of several other woman who said they felt a "spark" when they conceived.)

I had a very healthy pregnancy, as I knew I would. I vomited only one day during the entire nine months. I gave myself belief suggestions that I wasn't afraid of pregnancy, birth, and motherhood, and I never vomited again.

I kept exercising and continued to eat whatever I wanted (fruit, vegetables M&Ms, hamburgers, etc.), trusting that I knew what my body needed. I dreamt that I should continue to lift weights moderately, but that I should stop running—so I did.

I also dreamt frequently of giving birth. In the beginning of my pregnancy, I dreamt of giving birth in a hospital, surrounded by my father and other doctors. I was afraid and in pain. I gave myself suggestions that I wasn't afraid and that I believed in my ability to have a safe, easy birth at home. Soon my dreams reflected my beliefs.

After the pregnancy test I never returned to a doctor. David and I decided we would deliver the baby ourselves. We assumed I would go into some sort of altered state of consciousness and that the baby would be born easily.

I read Ina May Gaskin's *Spiritual Midwifery* (1978), which I found helpful for its description of labor as well as its birth stories from women on The Farm, a spiritual community in Tennessee. Although Ina May wouldn't have agreed, we decided our only tools would be a pair of scissors and a string.

Needless to say, my family thought we were nuts. My father told me I was literally insane. I had waited until I was seven months pregnant before telling them about it because I knew they weren't going to react well. I had seen them when I was six months along; my mother looked at me and said it was too bad I had gained back the weight I had lost. Basically, I didn't look pregnant. I just looked fat.

When I finally told them I was pregnant, my father said it was probably a psychological pregnancy. When they saw me again and faced up to the reality of the situation, my mother called Social Services in hopes they could convince me to change my mind about having an unassisted birth. A social worker and a visiting nurse stopped by periodically for the remainder of my pregnancy, with offers of help. We spoke with them openly about our beliefs, but I never allowed the nurse to examine me.

One night after wondering about the position of the baby, I dreamt that I saw it inside me, upside-down and ready to go. The next day I got a letter from my sister Susan, who at the time was a nurse working with women who had problems in labor (!). "How do you know if the baby's in the right position?" she asked frantically. It seemed as if everyone was worried except David and I. Our confidence in ourselves had grown right along with the baby. We knew we had help, but it was inner help and it was all the help we needed.

On the afternoon of August 20, 1978, I was walking back from the bookstore when I began feeling what I thought might be the beginning of labor. That night after dinner, I sat down and reread *Spiritual Midwifery*. My contractions were mild, so David and I decided to try and get some sleep. He slept; I didn't. Around midnight I got up and saw that I had lost my mucous plug. David changed the sheets and called some friends of ours who wanted to be at the birth. Three friends came over (all of them men, one of them a former boyfriend) along with a man who was making a film about us. I took a shower, sat down on the toilet (where my bowel emptied itself naturally), and basically stayed there for the next hour.

Everyone hung out with me in the bathroom, and we laughed thinking about how strange it must have looked—a woman in labor sitting on a toilet surrounded by five men. The mood was definitely that of a party, rather than a serious medical event. Everyone, including me, was having a good time.

After I lost my mucous plug, there was never any sense of a contraction starting, peaking, and ending, as I've read about in other women's births—just a general feeling of tightness. David had me say some belief suggestions that I wasn't afraid and that I believed in myself. I remember feeling, at one point, like a wild animal. I knew that my body knew exactly what it was doing.

Around 1:30 my water bag broke as I was sitting on the toilet. A minute later I reached down and felt the baby's face pressing against my perineum. I wasn't pushing. He was coming out on his own. I remember a friend had told me to be careful not to have the baby on the toilet, so I got up and held the baby's face as I walked over to the bed. I was on my hands and knees, about to turn over, when I heard a voice inside my head say, *"Don't turn over."* Since I hadn't read anything during my pregnancy about the undesirability of giving birth lying down, I had just assumed I would be on my back for the birth. There was no mistaking the intent of that voice, however, so I didn't turn over. A second later the baby came literally flying out of me. He felt so tiny my first thought was, *"Could that be the baby?"* (He was just under six pounds.) Reasoning instantly that it couldn't be anything else (!), I called out, "The Baby!" and David caught him in midair. I could feel the joy in his voice when he said, "It's a boy!"

He gave a little cry and someone helped me turn over. I remember being somewhat confused as I tried to decide which leg to lift up over the cord. David laid the baby on my belly. The little one was so still and peaceful that I asked, "Is he alive?" Everyone assured me he was fine. For the first time this baby was a reality to me. Somehow the whole pregnancy had seemed like a dream or a child's game. But this was real. A real live baby was lying on my belly.

After the cord stopped pulsating, our friend Rick tied a string around it and cut it with his pocket knife. Then all the men took the baby into the other room and gave him a bath. A few minutes later they brought him back in and he started to nurse.

About an hour and a half later I got up and went to the bathroom. The placenta slid into the toilet. One of the men retrieved it, put it in a plastic bag, and took it out to the woods nearby. Gradually everyone went home. David and I went to sleep with our little one between us.

The next few days were wonderful. I was a little sore because I had torn slightly, but I healed quickly. (Thinking back, I was probably a little too inhibited—with all those people around—to allow myself to relax totally. Still, I'm glad they were there because I felt at the time that I needed outside emotional support.) We decided to name the baby John because it was simple and unpretentious. In those days, people were naming their babies October Snow and Rainbow, so we thought we'd go in the opposite direction.

John was a beautiful baby and we loved just putting him between us and watching him sleep. Life was beautiful. We had been successful in creating the birth we desired. We were ready to take on the world. Little did we know, that was just what we were about to do.

Five days after John was born, we decided to call Fern, the visiting nurse, and invite her over to see the new baby. She and Jan, the social worker, came over and listened as we talked about how wonderful the birth had been. Fern asked if she could watch me nurse John. I agreed; and as I nursed, she wrote something down in the little notebook she sometimes carried. Then she and Jan left. Everything seemed to be going well. Several hours later though, Fern returned to say she wanted us to let a doctor examine John. He seemed perfect to us, so we refused.

That evening I was baking a cake when Fern, Jan, and three policemen banged on our door. They informed us that they were taking John. Fern thought he looked too thin, and they were taking him to the hospital to be examined.

Jan and Fern turned out to be from the child protection division of Social Services. They had been visiting us all along with the idea that anyone who would choose to have a baby at home, unassisted, was mentally deranged. As they carted John away, Jan informed us that he was now legally in the custody of the County Department of Social Services. David and I were horrified.

They let us come to the hospital, where a doctor glanced at John briefly and said, "It's obvious this child has been neglected." He was dehydrated, they said, and would need to be hospitalized for several days so he could receive fluids intravenously. They also said he was jaundiced and needed to be placed under bilirubin lights. (I've since learned that more than half of all babies are jaundiced within the first few days of life. Generally the condition clears up on its own.)

Apparently, when Fern had watched me nurse John she had written down, "Nursing improperly."

"Why didn't you just tell me?" I cried to her later.

"I didn't think you would listen," she replied.

Jan told us we could come back the next day and see John, but she was considering putting him in a foster home as soon as he recovered. According to her, we were, "psychologically disturbed."

David and I left the hospital in a state of shock. How could they even dream of putting John in a foster home? Couldn't they see how much we loved him?

That night when we returned to our little apartment filled with baby clothes and diapers, it was almost too much to bear. Could they really take him away from us? A day earlier we would have said, "Of course not!" But now everything seemed to be completely out of our control.

We both managed to calm down enough to fall asleep, only to have our respective nightmares.

David dreamt that he had gone to the hospital, but that policemen were standing in his way and they refused to let him see John. I dreamt I went to my parents' house and my father handed me a piece of paper. He said, "These are my rules and you are going to lived by them. Now sign this." I dutifully signed.

I awoke feeling worse than I had felt the night before. Yes, we felt liked victims. But here was a dream that vividly showed me signing over my own power, signing away my life.

David and I cried and yelled at each other for several hours. We knew we had gotten ourselves into this—but how could we get ourselves out? Legally, John wasn't even ours anymore. Suddenly I felt for all the parents who had ever lost a child. Whether by death or by physical separation, there is no greater pain.

At that moment I knew I had to decide whether I was going to go along with my father and the rest of officialdom, give up my power, and declare myself psychologically disturbed, or truly believe in myself and get my child back. "Fuck officialdom!" I yelled, "I'm not letting them take him away from us!"

David had done many rebellious things in his life, but I had always been a "good girl." So the decision to steal John from the hospital in a gym bag was a major step for me. We would "go on the lam," we decided. We would move from town to town if necessary. No one was taking our baby. Suddenly the whole thing turned into a great adventure—quite a change from the quiet life I had led as a doctor's daughter growing up in the suburbs.

We would only take him, we decided, if it looked as if they would actually put him in a foster home. He was our son, and no one was more qualified to raise him than we were. Ideally, of course, we wanted to believe that our belief in ourselves was strong enough so that we wouldn't have to carry out our plan. At that point, however, our faith had been shaken and we weren't taking any chances.

That afternoon I took my little blue gym bag and drove to the hospital. As I drove along the highway I was crying and literally screaming belief suggestions that I would be able to nurse John successfully and that he wouldn't be taken away from us.

My parents met me at the hospital. "Why don't you come home?" my mother said in a rare nurturing tone. "You can sit on the porch and I'll fix you something to eat."

"No," I replied. The temptation to give it all up and return to the "security" of my parents and officialdom was still too great. It was time to be brave and stand my ground.

I went into a small room at the hospital to lie down for a while. After twenty-four hours of total fear and anxiety, I felt strangely peaceful. It was as if I had become as stressed out as was spiritually and biologically possible and had fallen over an emotional waterfall into a sea of tranquillity. Jan came into the room. They would let us have John back if we agreed to allow them to come by periodically and counsel us. "Anything!" I said. "Just let us have him back!"

The next few days I pumped my breasts so the nurses could give John a bottle when I wasn't there. A kind nurse worked with me for a few minutes—and for the first time, John really latched onto my nipple.

After spending five days in the hospital, John came home. It was the happiest day of my life. Never again would I take anyone or anything for granted.

David and I continued to analyze everything that had happened to us. Fern gave us *The Tender Gift: Breastfeeding* (1976) by Dana Raphael, M.D.; and that helped shed some light on the situation.

We learned that, without emotional support, breast feeding is often difficult if not impossible. When I was pregnant, David had encouraged me to contact the La Leche League, in lieu of a supportive mother or female friend. I had refused out of fear they too would criticize me for having an unassisted birth.

We decided that this lack of support—coupled with some beliefs I still clung to at that time, concerning shame of my sexuality and bodily functions—is probably what caused me to have problems nursing. If my mother, Fern, and Jan could have put aside their fears and supported me in my decision to have an unassisted birth, I think my chances of nursing John would have been better. Even after he became dehydrated, I think I could have nursed him back to health with a little bit of help. Social Services, however, decided I needed to be taught a lesson. And I, in my ignorance, had obviously agreed.

When John was a few weeks old, David got a job at a recycling center and I began babysitting. Our lives were peaceful again—almost. Jan continued to "visit" us. Legally, Social Services had only given us temporary custody of John. Jan was to evaluate us; and when John was five months old, we were to go before a judge. The issue was not whether John would be put into a foster home. They were willing to let us keep him—as long as we submitted to ongoing psychiatric treatment. My desperate statement in the hospital about agreeing to "anything" was starting to haunt me. Jan was beginning to get very nosey in her periodic home visits.

When her questions turned to my sex life with David, I'd had enough.

"First of all," I said, "I don't think that's any of your business. Secondly, how can I feel comfortable telling you anything when I know you can use it against me in court?"

"Oh, don't worry about that," she reassured me. "All of this is confidential. I can't use it in court. I just want to help you."

I had learned not to trust this woman, so I continued to confine our conversations to neutral subjects.

Meanwhile, David and I tried to go on with our lives with the shadow of a court case hanging over our heads. Why, we wondered, were we putting ourselves through this? As much as we believed in ourselves, did we also believe that we were crazy? Were we going to court so that we would be forced to take a stand?

Fern continued to visit us separately. She had come to see that we were not crazy and was willing to put in a good recommendation for us in court—until one fateful day.

David and I had read in Dana Raphael's book that men were biologically capable of producing milk. David had no desire actually to nurse John, but he wanted to see if he could lactate simply by believing he could. He suggested to himself that he would produce milk—and within a week, one breast swelled up and milk began dripping out. My father looked at it briefly and said, "Obviously there's something physiologically wrong with David." The fact that David had mentally suggested this would happen was just a coincidence, in my father's mind.

Anyway, when Fern was just about to walk out the door one day, I stopped her. "Wait," I said. "I want to show you something." Reluctantly, David lifted up his shirt. He still didn't trust her. From the look on her face I knew I had made a mistake.

January 31, 1979, we went to court. On their side they had Jan, Fern, a psychiatrist we had never met, and the doctor who had said that John was neglected.

On our side we had a pediatrician we had been taking John to periodically on the advice of our lawyer. Of course, at that point we also had a firm belief that we would win.

Their doctor took the stand first and said that David had not been friendly to him that first night at the hospital. "He called me a 'pompous asshole,' " he said indignantly. Laughter filled the room, as it was obvious that David was right.

The psychiatrist took the stand and proceeded to analyze why I chose to have my baby at home without a doctor or midwife. "Her father is a physician," he said, "and obviously this was an act of rebellion." He also said that, in his opinion, both David and I were either socially unaware, psychotic, or had organic brain syndrome!

"Have you ever met these people?" the judge interjected.

"Well, no," he replied. With that, the judge ordered that his testimony be thrown out of court.

Fern took the stand and said that David wanted to lactate.

At last, Jan took the stand and said that David read books by seventeenth-century philosophers and thought that much of their knowledge had been lost by this society. This seemed to be a big deal to her. She had also mentioned it in her deposition. The statement itself didn't bother me, but she had learned about David's interest in seventeenth-century philosophers in one of our so-called confidential conversations at our apartment.

"Did you ever tell Laura and David that nothing they told you in your home visits could be used against them in court?" our lawyer asked. Jan answered with something totally unrelated. Our lawyer posed the question again, and again she avoided answering him. After she avoided the question five times, finally the judge stepped in.

"Just answer the question," he said. "Did you ever make that statement?"

"No," she replied. It was obvious that she was lying.

Our pediatrician took the stand and said that she felt David and I were good parents. We seemed emotionally stable and John was a healthy, happy baby. David and I were prepared to take the strand, but, our lawyer said it wasn't necessary. The judge threw the case out of court and told Social Services not to bother us again. David and I breathed a sigh of relief, left the courtroom, and went home confident that no one could ever stop us from creating the life we desired.

David stopped working at the recycling center after breaking an ankle and never went back. He had wanted to quit, but hadn't felt good about it. The ankle ended up being the excuse he felt he needed at the time.

He divided his time between reading books at the campus library and helping me take care of John and several other children we were babysitting for. We both continued to analyze ourselves, examine our dreams, and work on our bodies.

John was a healthy baby. He grew quickly and lived strictly off my breast milk until he was a year old. A woman at the recreation center where I worked out said to me when John was about nine months old, "You know, I'm a nurse and I can tell you for a fact that breast milk has no nutritional value for a baby after he's six months old."

"Gee," I said, "then shouldn't he be dead by now?" I had learned not to listen to so-called or self-proclaimed experts.

Another woman said to me, "Don't pick your baby up every time he fusses. You'll spoil him. He's got to learn he can't get whatever he wants in life." John rarely fussed because I rarely put him down. I kept him in his Snugli (front pack) as much as possible. I vacuumed with him in it as well as did my grocery shopping and anything else that I could. Not only did it keep him happy, but it also made me stronger.

At night he slept in between David and me and never cried when he was hungry. We had read in *The Tender Art: Breastfeeding* that babies only cry when they're hungry if their mother doesn't respond to the smacking noise they first make with their lips. A baby whose mother is down the hall and never hears the smacking noise will eventually stop making it and simply cry as soon as he is hungry. John was always within a few feet of either David or me, so he never had to resort to crying.

John never had diaper rashes or cried when he was cutting teeth. Because he was breast fed, and not bottle fed, he rarely spat up milk. When he did begin to eat solid food, we never resorted to the standard glass jars. We took turns chewing our food and giving it to him in little mouthfuls. I couldn't have asked for an easier baby.

The three of us were a happy little family. But still, we were isolated. My relationship with my parents had deteriorated after John's birth. They saw themselves as John's saviors, and we saw them as people who had tried to take our baby away from us. I didn't feel capable of having a relationship with either one of my sisters because I associated them with my parents.

David's mother lived in Texas, and his father had died when he was a teenager. Several years later, David's only brother had died of a drug overdose. Elva, his stepmother, lived nearby and was helpful financially and emotionally to a degree; but she still found our beliefs a little too strange to accept. "Why does David spend his days reading books?" she used to ask. "Why doesn't he go out and get a job like everyone else? Why doesn't he cut his hair and put on a suit and tie?"

No one, it seemed, understood our desire to withdraw from society for a while and concentrate on overcoming our psychological problems. Our thought at that time was, *"If we can work on ourselves for a while, eventually we can come back out into the world and be productive members of society."*

Of course, we never again wanted to be members of the suit-and-tie, conform-for-the-sake-of-conforming society. We pictured ourselves becoming a part of a new society. One that encouraged people to pursue their dreams whether that meant starting a business, reading a book, taking care of a child, or painting a picture.

Our lives, we decided, needed no justification. David didn't have to prove he was a real man by getting a job or fighting in a war. He was acceptable just the way he was. "Get out of the 60s," people used to say. "This is the real world and you have a family to support."

Somehow, we decided, we were going to support ourselves without compromising our beliefs. I was going to stay with John, and David was going to keep reading his books because that's what we wanted to do.

So, we started finding all kinds of ways to make money that were fun and creative. Our apartment was near some fraternity and sorority houses, and every few days John and I would walk down the alleys and see what treasures lay in or near the dumpsters. I always found books that I could sell to the used bookstore up the street. Once I found an antique doll; and another time, some old sheet music from the 1920s.

When one of the fraternities remodeled its house, all of the old furniture was thrown out. I took it up to the used furniture store; the money that it brought fed us for a week.

One night, as I was walking home from the store, I saw a man run into a parked car and then drive away. I got his license plate number and then put a note with my phone number on the windshield of the parked car. The man who owned the car was extremely appreciative and ended up giving me the car. It was old, but I found someone to buy it.

Once a man I knew told me to take as many apples as I wanted from his trees. I made apple pies periodically and traded them to the local pizza parlor for pizzas. One way or another, we always made it. We certainly weren't wealthy, but we decided long ago that wealth was not going to be a priority for us. We knew it would come eventually, however, if we kept working on ourselves psychologically.

Early in 1980 I realized I was pregnant. Once again I had a healthy pregnancy—never an ache or pain, and this time no vomiting at all. John continued to nurse and never seemed to care that my milk had disappeared.

I was planning on giving birth on my hands and knees because that had worked so well with John. But in a dream I was shown otherwise. In the dream, I was watching a woman deliver her own baby as she stood over a baby's bathtub—one of those little plastic tubs. I heard a woman's voice say to me gently, *"Tell her to remember not to do too much."* I understood what the woman meant, and the peaceful feeling of the dream stayed with me for the remainder of my pregnancy.

Around 7:30 in the morning on August 17, I began feeling some mild contractions. David and I made love, and I remember feeling an orgasm followed immediately by a contraction. They felt remarkably similar, but I must admit that the orgasm was more pleasant. I nursed John for a while and decided to take a shower. John was a little fussy and I felt maybe it would be better if I didn't wash my hair at that point.

I got out of the shower and was walking across the room when my water bag broke. It had been about two hours since my first contraction. I took out the little plastic bathtub and stood over it with my knees slightly bent as I had been shown in the dream. I didn't feel any more contractions after my water bag broke, but I knew I was having them because, when I put my hand up inside my vagina, I could feel my muscles rhythmically opening and closing around it.

A minute later a foot appeared between my legs. I wasn't expecting a breech birth, although a friend of mine had dreamt that he saw the baby inside me, standing up.

John pointed to the foot and asked, "What's that?"

"The baby's foot," I said.

David and I looked at each other. He looked a little worried. "What should we do?" he said. I assured him that everything was fine and that the baby would come out easily. In my calmest voice I said, "Look at me. Do I look worried?"

"Well, no," David replied.

Something went through my mind along the lines of, "*He bought it*"—because I actually was a little nervous. But I was determined to have this birth go smoothly.

David and I said some belief suggestions as the baby pointed its toes and wiggled its foot around as if it were testing water. With every contraction its foot got lower. I was actually finding it easier than John's birth because there was no pressure from the head.

About five minutes later, David and John went into the other room for some reason, and something inside me said the time was right. I gave one push, the other foot appeared, and in one smooth movement I grabbed both feet and pulled the baby out. David must have come back in at that point because I heard him say, "You did it!"

It was another boy. He gave a little cry and immediately started nursing. A few minutes later I delivered the placenta into the plastic bathtub. There was not a single sheet and only a couple of towels to wash—minor point perhaps but it was just one nice thing about the birth.

That afternoon we walked up to the corner grocery store and put the baby on the fruit scale: six pounds right on the nose. On our way home the name Willie popped into my head, and it seemed to fit him well. (Incidentally, twelve years after Willie's birth, I read in Janet Balaskas' *Active Birth* (1992:131) that, with a footling breech birth, it is absolutely essential for the mother to deliver in a "standing squat" position.)

About a week later I had a dream in which Willie told me that he had helped in the birth by not putting up any resistance from his end. A sort of tragi/comic image came into my mind of a baby in the womb saying sternly, "*I'm not coming out!*" Many people are willing to admit that a woman's attitude plays a big part in her labor, but few seem to consider the fact that perhaps the baby's attitude does, as well. Of course, even before birth, the baby is learning about life from the mother; so, her fear becomes his fear.

Willie was another peaceful little baby. Basically, he lived in a little "bouncey chair," as we used to call it. It was a reclining chair on a thick wire frame. We would rest a foot on it and give an occasional push, and Willie would bounce away contentedly for hours. Both the boys nursed and I had plenty of milk. Other than an occasional runny nose, they were very healthy.

When Willie was four months old, our landlord told us we would have to move. Our family was getting too large for a one-bedroom apartment. With $250 to our name I went out to find us a new place to live.

All the ads in the paper said, "First and last months' rent plus damage deposit," but somehow I figured I would get around that. I found a nice two-bedroom apartment for $350 a month. I told the landlady I had $250 and would get the rest to her within two weeks. I noticed she had three children so I said I would babysit off the damage deposit. She agreed and we moved in. I always managed to find neighborhood children to babysit for, as well. And so, the money kept coming in.

Every morning, David and I talked about our dreams, so the boys grew up believing that dreams and dream messages are just a normal part of life. John began telling us about his dreams almost as soon as he could talk. He never seemed to have frightening ones. I remember telling him once to go "pee-pee" before we went somewhere. He said he didn't have to because he went pee-pee in dreamland. Often he would talk about a "wreck" he visited in the mountains. He claimed there was some sort of treasure there.

David and I continued to use our dreams to gain insights into our daily lives. Once when I had a pain in my stomach that persisted for several weeks, I suggested to myself I would have a dream that would help me. That night I dreamt someone handed me a piece of paper, and the paper said, "*Here is why you're in pain, and here is what you can do to heal yourself.*"

The paper said I was hurting myself in an attempt to make Ed, our roommate at the time, feel sorry for me. Ed was in the process of moving out, and the paper explained that I thought maybe I could get him to stay by making myself out to be pitiful.

My "feel sorry for me" complex was something I had been aware of in the past, but I didn't realize that I still clung to it. The paper went on to say that I should direct my energies into improving my relationship with David, and just let Ed go. I did, and the pain disappeared the following day.

Little by little, David and I were seeing that we really could create happy, healthy lives for ourselves by working with our beliefs.

In the summer of 1982 I realized I was pregnant again. David and I were enjoying our family, and our only real concern was money. We always had enough to pay the bills, but nothing more. We trusted, however, that more money would come in by the time the baby arrived.

When I was eight months pregnant, a friend suggested we sell donuts door to door in the university dorms. I suggested we sell them to the university itself, and let the *school* sell them one by one. She didn't like my idea, so I decided to do it on my own.

I went to the local donut shop and asked if I could take samples up to the university. They said yes and encouraged me to take them to other businesses around town, as well.

When I talked to the head of food service at the university, he said, "Just today we decided to start taking donuts in the dorms. We'll take five hundred dozen a week."

I hired a driver and rounded up a few more accounts. Then, with my stomach bulging and kids in tow, I headed down to the next small city, and convinced the big brewery there to buy from me, as well. Soon I had a thriving little business. I was glad the new source of money arrived before the baby did.

On the morning of November 16, David left for the library and I went into labor. We had decided that, if David happened to be there, I wouldn't ask him to leave; but ideally I wanted to do this one alone. I had come to see birth as a personal challenge, and I was confident I was up to the task.

I informed the boys that the baby was coming soon, but then nothing happened. If someone called or came over, I felt contractions. But as soon as I was by myself, they would stop. Still, I wanted to go through with my plan.

My friend Laurie took me and the boys to the park, and I tried to relax. I seemed to go in and out of labor all day.

The next morning, David left for the library again and my contractions started picking up. The boys were still sleeping, and I decided to take a shower. Although there had been some slightly uncomfortable contractions with both Willie and John, this time the contractions were causing me some pain. I knew it was because I was afraid to be alone, so I said some belief suggestions and reassured myself that I was only alone physically.

When I got out of the shower, I took out my little plastic bathtub and washed my scissors and string with hot water. The phone rang. It was the secretary at the university wanting to give me a donut order.

"I'm in labor right now," I said. "Can I call you back in a couple of hours?"

Frantically she said, "But who am I going to give this order to?!"

I had to laugh. She seemed more concerned with getting her order out than I was with getting my baby out. "I really will call you back," I said, and hung up the phone.

A few minutes later, I straddled the bathtub and got down on one knee—the position that felt right for me this time. The baby started coming out and I saw my water bag break over her face. She looked straight up at me and cried. The joy that I felt at that moment was beyond description. The thought went through my mind that she was the most beautiful gift I had ever received. ("Weren't we beautiful, too?" the boys later asked. Of course they were. But for some reason, that was the thought in my mind at the time.)

I wrapped her up in a towel and put her in the bouncey chair while I delivered the placenta into the tub. Then I tied and cut the cord and went over to the couch to lie down for a while. The boys woke up and were excited to have a new little sister. John made me a glass of chocolate milk, and it tasted wonderful.

As I lay there, the sound of ocean waves and soft bells filled my head. I felt absolutely blissful. After about an hour and a half, I got up, took a shower, and got dressed. I dressed Joy (as we decided to call her) and put her in a little white wicker doll carriage that had been Elva's as a child. Then we all walked over to the campus to see David.

It was a beautiful day. The temperature was in the seventies and I felt positively high. This, I thought, must be what Grantly Dick-Read meant when he wrote that childbirth gives a woman a feeling of exaltation.

When I got over to the campus, some friends of David said he had gone home, so I called him on the phone and told him he had a daughter. He said he knew the baby had been born because he saw the placenta in the tub.

David walked back over to meet us and joined me, Joy, the boys, and our friends in celebrating the birth of our first little girl.

Not everything was glorious in those days. David struggled with minor health problems, and both of us had to deal with periodic bouts of depression. After Ed moved out, we had few visitors. The donut business kept us going, but we had no money to take vacations or even go out to dinner. We enjoyed our children and told ourselves that eventually things would change for us. Someday our beliefs would not cause us to be social outcasts. And someday we would have the money to go more places and do more things.

In the meantime, David was committed to reading his books, which at that time dealt with everything from politics to psychology, and I was committed to being with the kids.

In the spring of 1984 I realized that once again I was pregnant. I hadn't used any birth control since 1977 because I believed, or thought I believed, that I could control my own body. We had always said we wanted a large family, but money was now becoming a big problem. If only I could be as proficient at creating money as I was at creating babies. We knew we still had mental blocks concerning money, and we were trying our best to deal with them. We certainly didn't need the pressure of another mouth to feed.

My dreams showed me that, as far as money was concerned, I was keeping it from coming to me out of fear that it would somehow destroy me. My father's partner's wife had committed suicide when I was a teenager. They were wealthy, by my standards; and somehow I had decided that wealth led to unhappiness. In a dream I found myself saying that I didn't want money because I didn't want to end up like Mrs. Huttner.

Of course, the myth of the "happy poor" was certainly pushed by corporate America when I was growing up. The TV Waltons were poor but happy, while the more affluent members of society were turning into alcoholics and getting divorced. Some part of me had bought that myth as easily as many people in my parents' generation had bought the myth that *all* one needed to be happy were money and status.

Other dreams showed me why I was obsessed with pregnancy. In one, I was being chased by someone who wanted to hurt me. I turned to him and said, "*You can't hurt me. I'm pregnant.*" The man turned and walked away. Obviously, pregnancy made me feel less vulnerable. Women are often thought of as sluts and whores. But mothers are sacred, especially when they are pregnant.

Besides, if I was nothing else, I was a good birther. Giving birth was the one thing in my life that had given me any sense of accomplishment. But now I needed to direct my energies into taking care of the children I had.

I said belief suggestions that I would miscarry, but nothing happened. I didn't want to get an abortion because I was too afraid and because, at that time, I looked on abortion as an admission of failure. So, David and I decided to make the best of it.

About five weeks before I thought the baby would be born, I had a dream that I saw a woman giving birth. Someone said, "*She finally let go of the baby.*" The next morning I went into labor. Rather than admitting I was going into labor prematurely, I told myself that perhaps I had miscalculated my due date.

David had already left for the library, and the kids were still asleep. I decided to take a bath. After soaking for a while, I stood up and my water bag broke. I noticed that there was meconium in the amniotic fluid. Seconds later, the baby slid out into my hands. He was blue and lifeless. I breathed into his nose and mouth and he began crying. He nursed a little and looked content, but a few hours later he simply closed his eyes and died. David had come home right after the birth and was the one who noticed the baby died. I assumed he was just sleeping.

We called the paramedics. And as they tried to bring the life back into his tiny body, I was torn between wanting him to live and knowing somehow it would be better if he didn't.

He was gone. The coroner said he had a congenital heart defect, influenza, pneumonia, and basically an infection of the entire body. We grieved for him but knew this was just not the right time for him to be here.

A few days later a man whose wife was pregnant and planning on delivering in the hospital (the "right" way) said to me, "So are they going to put you in jail now?" To this day, I think it was the most insensitive remark anyone has ever made to me. I was horrified. I called the coroner and asked him if he felt I was responsible for my baby's death. "No," he said, "the baby just didn't develop the body to survive."

Several years before, my father's sister had given birth to a baby with a heart defect. That baby was kept alive on a respirator for several months before he finally died. Still, some people blamed me for my baby's death. Everyone who was looking for a reason not to take us seriously finally had one. "We knew it would happen eventually," they said.

In time, however, we came to look on the baby's death as a blessing. We weren't ready for another baby. As cruel as it may sound to some people, for us his death was the manifestation of my desire to miscarry. It was just slow in coming.

In 1985 the donut business became too competitive and I gave it up. I got a job as a cocktail waitress and topless dancer at a bar not too far from my house. Joy was two and a half and I decided to wean her. (I had nursed the boys until age three.) For the first time, I had to leave my family, but it gave me a chance to explore another aspect of my personality. David took over most of the cooking, cleaning, and childcare. I often wondered who had the harder job.

The bar was a nice one, and the dancing wasn't too risqué. The emphasis was more on sensuality than sexuality. Some of the girls choreographed numbers from *Cabaret* or *Cats* and put a lot of time and effort into practicing. I had my own shows I put together, and I enjoyed performing. I used to imagine, when I was on stage, that I was confronting my grade school principal who had insisted on "proper attire." "How's this?!" I would yell as I threw off my bra. I soon learned to feel very comfortable without my clothes on.

The money was better than it had been in the donut business, and the exercise was great for my body. In a sense, I felt I was reliving my adolescence. I flirted with men and was showered with attention—something I wasn't able to experience when I actually was an adolescent.

At the end of 1986 I realized that, yes, I was pregnant again. It had been more than two years since my last pregnancy, and I thought I had become quite proficient at mental birth control. We had moved into a four-bedroom house that Elva had helped us buy; so, space wasn't a problem. But could we really afford another child? The kids were four, six, and eight; and David and I missed having a little one around. Still, we were hesitant. So I went to an abortion clinic and had an ultrasound done. I found out I was more than three months along and that the placenta had partially separated from the uterine wall.

"If you have this baby," the nurse said, "you'll probably bleed a lot when it's born." A nurse I worked with at the bar said, "The baby will probably be brain damaged because of the placental separation." I made an appointment to have an abortion the following week.

The next few days, David and I struggled with our decision. One night I woke up screaming. We wanted this baby, but some part of us felt it wasn't the "responsible" thing to do. David's mother wrote from Texas, "You're breeding like animals!" No one, it seemed, thought we should have this baby.

The day before I was scheduled to have the abortion, I called and canceled it. That night I felt the baby kick for the first time.

I stopped dancing, but continued to wait on tables. My money remained the same, and it felt good to stay active. I worked right up until the end.

On the Friday night of April 3, I finished my shift and went home to enjoy my weekend. Sunday morning around 7:00, I began feeling contractions. David got up and went out on the couch to read the paper. I didn't tell him I was in labor. I dozed off and on for an hour and gave myself suggestions that I was completely cooperating with my body. *"I'm not fighting this in any way,"* I told myself. *"I trust that my body knows exactly what it's doing."*

As I breathed deeply, I felt myself slip into a state of complete relaxation. There was not a tense muscle in my entire body. This was the state I had been striving for in my other births. At last, I had reached it. I actually fell asleep and had a dream, but couldn't remember what it was about when I woke up.

At 8:15 I got up, walked across the hall to the bathroom, and turned on the bathwater.

"You taking a bath?"David called out from the living room.

"Yes," I replied. I didn't feel like involving him at that point. I felt perfectly capable of handling it myself.

As the bathwater was running, I sat down on the toilet and noticed the water bag between my legs. Suddenly it popped and the baby's head appeared. I gave a little push and she slid out into my hands. The cord was wrapped loosely around her neck and I unwound it. She gave a little cry and immediately started nursing.

"David," I called out, "will you come here a minute?" David walked down the hall. He had heard the little cry, but thought there was a cat in the bathroom. He looked in, and his eyes widened as he saw Michelle sitting on my lap.

"You better get a scissors and string," I said, "and turn off the bathwater." Soon, I delivered the placenta (into the toilet, again), and David cut the cord. (This time we didn't bother to tie it.) Contrary to what the nurse had predicted, I hardly bled at all.

Some girls from work had scheduled a baby shower for me that afternoon. (I had thought the baby would be born around the middle of the month. Naturally, then, I hadn't objected when they wanted to have the shower on April 5.) I felt great—so, Joy, Michelle, Elva, and I went to the shower. Needless to say, the girls were surprised to see Michelle on the *outside* of my body. It was truly a day of celebration.

Conclusion

Each of my births was truly unique. However, there are many elements that were common to all of them.

DURING MY PREGNANCIES

- I examined my beliefs about birth and life in general.
- I looked for evidence of limiting beliefs that could possibly prevent me from having a good birth.
- I read books that dealt with the power of belief.
- I read Ina May Gaskin's *Spiritual Midwifery* (1978) during my first pregnancy. The book helped me to understand both the physical and spiritual aspects of birth.
- I visualized myself having the kind of birth I desired.
- I spent a lot of time with my husband.
- I avoided people who were not supportive of what I was doing.
- I analyzed my dreams. Moreover, in my dreams I practiced giving birth.
- I told myself daily that I wasn't fearful, shameful, or guilty; that I loved and forgave myself; and that I believed in my ability to give birth safely and easily.

- I ate whatever I wanted, which included meat, sugar, salt, fruit, vegetables, and anything else that looked appealing.
- I didn't get on a scale.
- I lifted weights, but stopped jogging when I was about three months pregnant.

WHILE IN LABOR

- I relaxed completely, breathed deeply, took a bath or shower, made love, ate, drank, slept, went to the bathroom, took walks, or nursed a child, all depending on my feelings at the time.
- I said my belief suggestions.
- I didn't time contractions or check to see how dilated I was.
- I got in the position that made me the most comfortable.
- I trusted that I had inner help.
- Other than a slight push or two in the last seconds of labor, I didn't push. I allowed the baby to come out when ready.
- Above all, as I had been instructed in the second-pregnancy dream, *I remembered not to do too much.*

AFTER THE BIRTHS

- I offered my breast to the baby.
- I wrapped the baby in a blanket or towel.
- I waited a few minutes before tying and cutting the cord.
- I tied a string around the cord about an inch from the belly button, and cut the cord just above it with a clean pair of scissors. (With Michelle's birth, we cut the cord without tying it. The healing took place just as quickly and easily as with the others.)
- I calmly waited for the placenta to slide out either into the toilet or bathtub. Generally this happened within minutes of the birth; but with the first one, it took over an hour.
- Other than with my first birth in which I had torn slightly, I began exercising the following day.

THE PRESENT

Today my children are six, eleven, thirteen, and fifteen. David and I have raised them in the same spirit in which they were birthed. We've taught them to believe in themselves completely and not fear themselves or their world.

They all do well in school. However, we've never pushed them to excel academically. Above all, we wanted them to enjoy their childhood.

For the most part, they get along well with each other. They have numerous friends and are well liked by their teachers. They've always been healthy; and this past year, all four of them had perfect attendance in school.

David and I believe that their peaceful births, coupled with the love and attention we have always given the children, has contributed greatly to their happy, well-balanced personalities.

The following statement is from Barbara W. Spengler, a teacher who taught all four of them. I'm including it here not to show the superiority of my children, but to show the superiority of following nature's way.

I have had the pleasure of having all four of David and Laura Shanley's children in my classroom. There are many fine qualities that they all possess and I appreciated as a teacher. In the academic areas they are conscientious and dependable, but they are children who are willing to help others without being asked. They are self disciplined and know that it takes hard work to accomplish a goal. In group activities they are very cooperative and have excellent peer relationships. On an individual basis each one has his/her own personality. However, I also sense a great deal of family pride and love and a sincere respect for each other and their parents. In a time of many dysfunctional families, the Shanleys have brought into the world and are rearing four responsible, emotionally stable, caring children who I predict will carry these qualities into their adult life.

This past Christmas, David and I reconciled with our families. David saw his mother for the first time in twenty years, and we had the extreme pleasure of sharing our children with her. She has always "loved them from afar," but for the first time she was able to be with them physically.

Elva, David's stepmother, actually invited David's mother to stay at her house during the visit. There was never any sense of animosity between the two of them. They lovingly shared their grandchildren.

I called my parents on Christmas Day and went to see them several days later. After a few hours of tearful admissions of love and apologies on both sides, we took the children to the zoo. As we strolled along and gazed at the numerous Christmas lights decorating the trees and animal houses, my mother put her arm around me and said this was truly a "magical night." My sister Janet went with us, and she and the children took to each other right away. Several months later, my sister Susan and her family came to visit. We all had a wonderful time getting to know each other.

In April, David, the children, Elva, and I went to my parents' house for Passover dinner. I could see the joy and pride in my fathers' eyes as he watched the children read the prayers. Later I heard my mother say to my father, "I feel like we have our daughter back."

I think all of us learned, in those years of separation, how important family is. David and I understand now that not everyone in this world is going to agree with us. But that doesn't mean we have to isolate ourselves from the rest of humanity. We can be tolerant of other people's beliefs—and in turn, hopefully, they will be tolerant of ours.

I would like to end this book by quoting Grantly Dick-Read, a man who has inspired me both in birth and in life.

> If left alone in labor, the body of a woman produces most easily the baby that is not interfered with by its mother's mind or the assistant's hand. If left alone, just courage and patience are required. Faith, if she is a believer, is the secret of having a healthy baby and being a happy mother. (Dick-Read 1959:232)

Bibliography

Abbott, Karen. 1992a. "Cesarean Robs Mom of Birthing Experience." *Rocky Mountain News*, November 30.
———. 1992b. "Obstetricians Run Amuck." *Rocky Mountain News*, Denver, Colo., November 30.
Allen, James. 1993. *As a Man Thinketh*. Stamford, Conn.: Longmeadow Press.
Arms, Suzanne. 1975. *Immaculate Deception*. Boston: Houghton Mifflin.
Armstrong, Penny, and Sheryl Feldman. 1990. *A Wise Birth*. New York: William Morrow.
Bach, Richard. 1977. *Illusions*. New York: Dell Publishing.
Balaskas, Janet. 1992. *Active Birth*. Boston: Harvard Common Press.
Brackbill, Yvonne, June Rice, and Diony Young. 1984. *Birth Trap: The Legal Low-down on High-tech Obstetrics*. St. Louis: C. V. Mosby.
Bradley, Robert A. 1965. *Husband-coached Childbirth*. New York: Harper & Row.
———. 1967. *Psychic Phenomena: Revelations and Experiences*. West Nyack, N.Y.: Parker Publishing.
Caldeyro-Barcia, Roberto. 1975. "Supine Called the Worst Position for Labor and Delivery." *Family Practice News* 5:11.
Carter, Patricia Cloyd. 1957. *Come Gently, Sweet Lucina*. Titusville, Fla.: Patricia Cloyd Carter.
Cohen, Nancy, and Lois Estner. 1983. *Silent Knife: Cesarean Prevention and Vaginal Birth after Cesarean*. South Hadley, Mass.: Bergin & Garvey.

Corliss, William. 1982. *The Unfathomed Mind: A Handbook of Unusual Mental Phenomena*. Glen Arm, Md.: Sourcebook Project.

Davis-Floyd, Robbie E. 1992. *Birth as an American Rite of Passage*. Berkeley and Los Angeles: University of California Press.

————. 1993. "Hospital Birth as a Technocratic Rite of Passage." *Mothering*, no. 67 (Spring):68–75.

Delaney, Gayle. 1988. *Living Your Dreams*. San Francisco: Harper & Row.

Dick-Read, Grantly. 1959. *Childbirth without Fear: The Principles and Practice of Natural Childbirth*. New York: Harper & Row.

Dwinell, Jane. 1992. *Birth Stories: Mystery, Power, and Creation*. Westport, Conn.: Bergin & Garvey.

Eaton, S. Boyd, Marjorie Shostak, and Melvin Konner. 1988. *The Paleolithic Prescription*. San Francisco: Harper & Row.

Fletcher, Jan. 1988. "No More Professional Pushers." Your Letters section. *Mothering*, no. 49 (Fall):12.

Gaskin, Ina May. 1978. *Spiritual Midwifery*. Summertown, Tenn.: The Book Publishing Company.

————. 1987. "Childbirth the Amish Way." *Mothering*, no. 43 (Summer):70–71.

Goldsmith, Judith. 1990. *Childbirth Wisdom from the World's Oldest Societies*. Brookline, Mass.: East West Health Books.

Gossett, Don. 1976. *What You Say Is What You Get*. Springdale, Pa.: Whitaker House.

Haggard, Howard W., M.D. 1929. *Devils, Drugs, and Doctors*. New York: Harper & Row.

Haire, Doris. 1972. *The Cultural Warping of Childbirth*. Minneapolis: International Childbirth Education Association.

Harrison, Michelle. 1982. *A Woman in Residence*. New York: Random House.

Hartman, Ruth. 1993. "Changing Beliefs about Birth." *Boulder Parent*, Colorado (January):1–10.

Heard, Gerald. 1949. *Prayers and Meditations*. New York: Harper & Brothers.

————. 1963. *The Five Ages of Man*. New York: Julian Press.

Jacobson, B., G. Eklund, L. Hamberger, D., Linarsson, G. Sedvall, and M. Valvereius. 1987. "Perinatal Origin of Adult Self-destructive Behavior." *Acta Psychiatrica Scandinavica* 76:364–371.

Jones, Carl. 1987. *Mind over Labor*. New York: Penguin Books.

Kalichman, N., M.D. 1951. "On Some Psychological Aspects of the Management of Labor." *Psychiatric Quarterly* 25, no. 4:655.

Kitzinger, Sheila. 1979. *Birth at Home*. New York: Penguin Books.

Konner, Melvin. 1987. *Becoming a Doctor: A Journey of Initiation in Medical School*. New York: Viking.

Korte, Diana, and Roberta Scaer. 1990. *A Good Birth, A Safe Birth*. Boston, Mass.:Harvard Common Press.

Krauska, Patricia Corrigan. 1976. "Some Mothers Prefer Home Births." *St. Louis Globe Democrat*, January 15.

Ludivici, Anthony M. 1938. *The Truth about Childbirth*. New York: E. P. Dutton.

Mendelsohn, Robert S. 1979. *Confessions of a Medical Heretic*. Chicago: Contemporary Books.

Mitford, Jessica. 1992. *The American Way of Birth*. New York: Penguin Books U.S.A.

Moran, Marilyn A. 1981. *Birth and the Dialogue of Love*. Leawood, Kans.: New Nativity Press.

————. 1986. *Happy Birth Days*. Leawood, Kans.: New Nativity Press.

————. 1992. "Attachment or Loss within Marriage: The Effect of the Medical Model of Birthing on the Marital Bond of Love." *Pre- and Peri-natal Psychology Journal* 6, no. 4 (Summer):265–279.

————. 1993. "The Effect of Lovemaking on the Progress of Labor." *Pre - and Peri-natal Psychology Journal* 7, no. 3 (Spring):231–241.

Morris, Desmond. 1986. *Cat Watching*. New York: Crown Publishers.

Odent, Michel. 1992. *The Nature of Birth and Breastfeeding*. Westport, Conn.: Bergin & Garvey.

Peale, Norman Vincent. 1990. *The Power of Positive Living*. New York: Ballantine Books.

Peterson, Gayle. 1981. *Birthing Normally: A Personal Growth Approach to Childbirth*. Berkeley, Calif.: Mindbody Press.

Purina. 1981. *Handbook of Cat Care*. St. Louis, Mo.: Purina Cat Care Center.

Rank, Otto. 1952. *The Trauma of Birth*. New York: Brunner.

Raphael, Dana. 1976. *The Tender Gift: Breastfeeding*. New York: Schocken Books.

Roberts, Jane. 1970. *The Seth Material*. Englewood Cliffs, N.J.: Prentice-Hall.

————. 1972. *Seth Speaks: The Eternal Validity of the Soul*. Englewood Cliffs, N.J.: Prentice-Hall.

————. 1974. *The Nature of Personal Reality: A Seth Book*. New York: Prentice-Hall.

————. 1979. *The Nature of the Psyche: Its Human Expression*. New York: Prentice-Hall.

————. 1981. *The God of Jane: A Psychic Manifesto*. Englewood Cliffs, N.J.: Prentice-Hall.

Rocky Mountain News, Denver, Colo. 1992. "Quality of Ultrasound Tested." December 1, 1992.

Samuels, Mike, and Nancy Samuels. 1975. *Seeing with the Mind's Eye*. New York: Random House.

Sanford, John A. 1989. *Dreams: God's Forgotten Language*. San Francisco: Harper & Row.

Shearer, Beth. 1989. "Forced Cesareans: The Case of the Disappearing Mothers." *International Journal of Childbirth Education* 4, no. 1:7–10.

Siegel, Bernie S. 1986. *Love, Medicine, and Miracles*. New York: Harper & Row.

Sinetar, Marsha. 1990. *Living Happily Ever After: Creating Trust, Luck, and Joy*. New York: Villard Books.

Sousa, Marion. 1976. *Childbirth at Home*. Englewood Cliffs, N.J.: Prentice-Hall.

Stewart, David, and Lee Stewart, eds. 1981. *The Five Standards for Safe Childbearing*. Marble Hill, Mo.: NAPSAC.

Stukane, Eileen. 1985. *The Dream Worlds of Pregnancy*. New York: William Morrow.

Talbot, Michael. 1988. *Beyond the Quantum*. New York: Bantam Books.

————. 1991. *The Holographic Universe*. New York: Harper Perennial.

Tatje-Broussard, Nancy. 1990. "Second Stage Labor: You Don't Have to Push." *Mothering*, no. 57 (Fall):78–81.

Tew, Marjorie. 1990. *Safer Childbirth: A Critical History of Maternity Care*. New York: Routledge, Chapman, and Hall.

Ubell, Earl. 1993. "Are Births as Safe as They Could Be?" *Parade* magazine, February 7.

Wallis, Charles L. 1965. *The Treasure Chest*. New York: Harper & Row.

Webster's New Collegiate Dictionary. 1981. Springfield, Mass.: G. & C. Merriam.

Wessel, Helen S. 1963. *Natural Childbirth and the Christian Family*. New York: Harper & Row.

Windle, William F. 1969. "Brain Damage by Asphyxia at Birth." *Scientific American* (October):77–84.

Young, Diony, and Beth Shearer. 1987. "Crisis in Obstetrics: The Management of Labor." *C/Sec Newsletter* 13, no. 3.

Index

About the Author

LAURA KAPLAN SHANLEY is a free-lance writer who has contributed to journals and magazines on subjects of childbirth and spirituality.